Table of Contents

What is a very low carb/high fat lifestyle? 2

The science of carbohydrate 2

The science supporting a very low carb/high fat lifestyle 4

How could this lifestyle benefit me? 8

Not a quick fix but sustainable lifestyle change 9

Questions to ask yourself before you start 9

Step 1: What are you currently eating? 10

Step 2: Identification of carbohydrate foods 12

Step 3: Eliminating carbohydrates - how low do you go? 15

Step 4: What can you eat? 16

Step 5: Monitoring success 20

Step 6: Maintenance 31

Essential tips to ensure success e.g. eating enough salt and fat 32

Frequently asked questions 37

Filling up on fat 45

Focus on alcohol 50

Zero and low calorie sweeteners 52

Glycaemic Index 55

Reading and understanding food labels 56

Carbohydrate content of everyday foods 58

Sample meal plans 68

Low carb recipes 72

Where can I obtain further information and support? 78

Health indicators 79

Monitoring health 85

www.xperthealth.org.uk

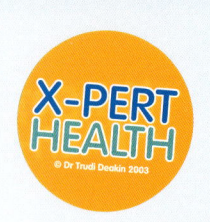

What is a very low carb/high fat lifestyle?

What is carbohydrate?
Carbohydrate is a nutrient found in starchy and sugary foods. There are four nutrients in the diet that provide calories: carbohydrate and protein contribute 4kcal per gram, fat provides 9kcal per gram, and alcohol 7kcal per gram. A low carbohydrate diet means that you reduce the amount of carbohydrate that you are eating and obtain your calories from the other nutrients.

Definitions for different amounts of carbohydrate in the diet

A high carbohydrate diet has been recommended for decades and therefore most people obtain around half of their daily calories (~50%) from carbohydrate. The reference intake (RI) for a healthy adult is set at 260g of carbohydrate per day, which is equal to 1,040 calories. Reference Intakes are not targets but they enable people to assess their diets to determine what dietary approach they are adopting.

A moderate carbohydrate diet contains 26 to 45% of calories from carbohydrate. This equates to between 130g and 225g of carbohydrate per day.

A low carbohydrate diet contains less than 130g per day or less than 26% total energy. This is the amount of glucose that the brain and central nervous system requires per day to function properly.

A very low carb/high fat lifestyle provides just 20 to 50g of carbohydrate per day or less than 10% of a 2000 kcal per day diet. At this level of carbohydrate restriction, the brain and central nervous system cannot obtain the 130g of glucose per day that it requires and therefore fat stores are broken down to produce chemicals called ketones. Ketones can supply the essential energy required for the brain reducing dependance on dietary carbohydrate.

The science of carbohydrate

What happens when we eat carbs? Carbohydrate (sugar and starch) is made from building blocks of glucose. During the process of digestion, carbohydrates break down releasing glucose, causing blood glucose levels to rise. The increase in blood glucose triggers the pancreas to release a hormone called insulin into the blood. This hormone acts like a key, unlocking the door into the body cells so that the glucose can pass from the blood into the body cell where it is either used for energy, stored as an energy reserve or converted to fat (see figure 1).

Why may I struggle to control my weight if I am having a high carbohydrate diet? Two out of three people have insulin resistance. This means that the insulin they release from the pancreas doesn't work as efficiently as it could i.e. it struggles to open the cell door and allow the glucose to enter the cell. The body responds to this by releasing extra insulin to do the job. This is usually successful at enabling the glucose to be cleared from the blood and normal blood glucose to be maintained between 4 and 7mmol/l.

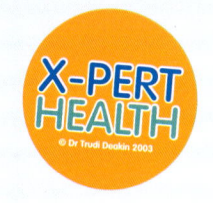

The science of carbohydrate

Figure 1: What happens when we eat carbs?

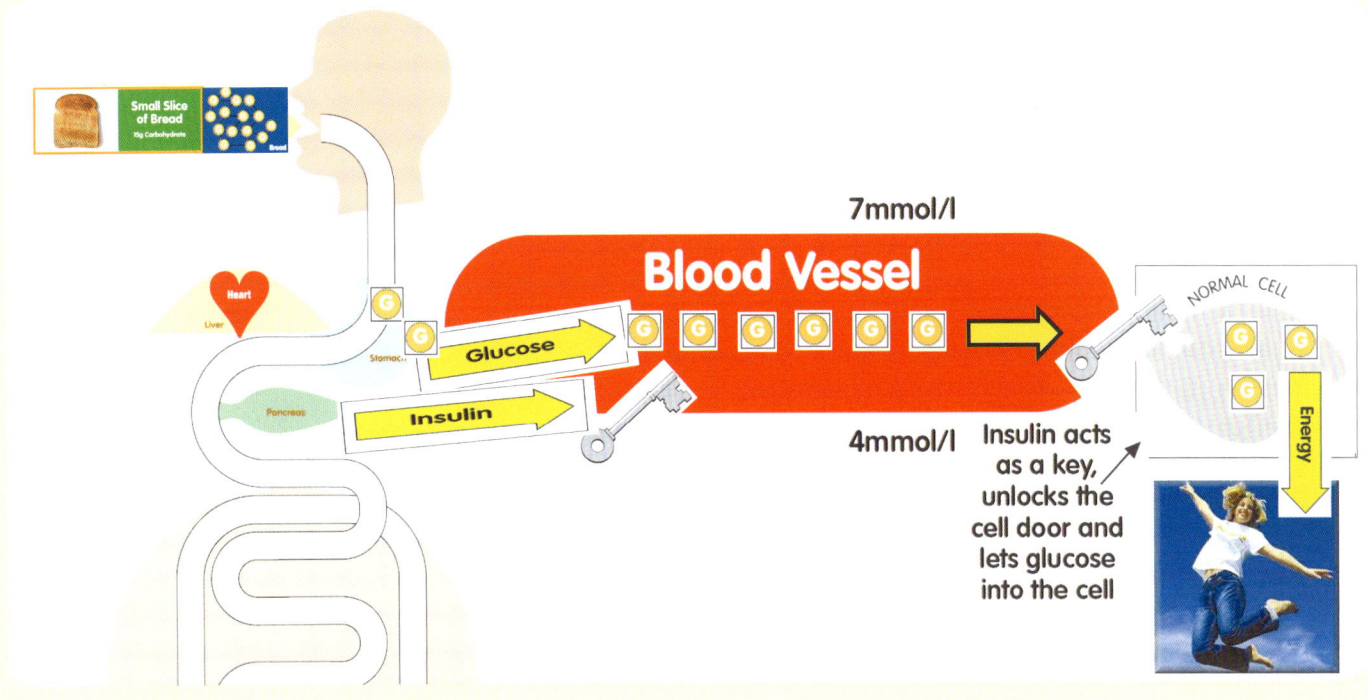

Insulin is what we call an anabolic hormone. This means that it is weight promoting by encouraging the production and storage of fat from carbohydrate. Therefore although it is good news that extra insulin is made to control blood glucose levels, it is bad news that weight gain or prevention of weight loss is experienced. If you currently base your meals around carbohydrate and struggle to maintain or lose weight, it may be that you have insulin resistance.

Is there a test for insulin resistance?

There are blood tests that can assess how much insulin you are producing and levels of insulin resistance but these are currently not included in the standard tests undertaken by your GP. However, if you have three or more of the following factors, it is likely that you have the metabolic syndrome and insulin resistance (see Health Indicators pages 79-84).

- Increased waist size: Caucasian men greater than 94 cm and women greater than 80 cm
  South Asian men greater than 90 cm and women greater than 80 cm
- Raised triglycerides: greater than 1·7 mmol/L (or on medication to reduce triglycerides)
- Reduced HDL-cholesterol (the good cholesterol): less than 1·03 mmol/L) in men; less than 1·29 mmol/L in women
- Raised blood pressure: Systolic greater than 130 mmHg; Diastolic greater than 85 mmHg (or on medication to reduce blood pressure)
- Raised fasting glucose: Fasting plasma glucose greater than 5·6 mmol/L

N.B. Most people with Type 2 diabetes will have the metabolic syndrome based on these criteria.

What is diabetes?

In some individuals, the additional insulin still doesn't manage to control blood glucose levels and in others, the pancreas becomes tired from making extra insulin and starts to slow down. In both cases this results in blood glucose levels rising above 7mmol/l and Type 2 diabetes is diagnosed. Type 1 diabetes is a different condition whereby the pancreas stops making insulin altogether and people have to start either injecting it or using an insulin pump.

www.xperthealth.org.uk

The science supporting a very low carb/high fat lifestyle

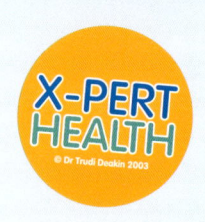

There is emerging evidence that a very low carb/high fat lifestyle has many health benefits

Health benefits shown in clinical studies

A reduction in:
- appetite
- prescribed medication
- risk of heart disease and stroke
- irritable bowel syndrome (IBS) symptoms
- premenstrual tension (PMT) symptoms
- C-reactive protein (a marker of inflammation and a risk factor for heart disease, diabetes & arthritis)
- oxidative stress and aging
- blood glucose levels
- blood pressure readings
- triglyceride levels (a type of fat in the blood)
- small dense LDL particles (the carriers of cholesterol that easily become oxidised causing fatty plaques that clog up the arteries)
- insulin resistance and insulin levels

Improvements in:
- weight loss and fat loss compared to low fat diets
- HDL cholesterol (which reduces the risk of heart disease and strokes)
- liver function
- acne and skin appearance
- heartburn and acid reflux
- polycystic ovarian syndrome

Possible treatment for:
- neurological and neurodegenerative diseases such as epilepsy, Alzheimer's, Parkinson's, Multiple Sclerosis and mental health disorders such as bipolar
- cancer (but work is in early stages and much more research is needed)

A reduction in appetite

The reason why most diets fail is due to hunger. Many people start to feel miserable and eventually give up on their diet. One of the best things about adopting the low carb high fat approach is that it leads to an automatic reduction in appetite. Studies consistently show that when people cut carbs and eat more fat they eat less frequently.

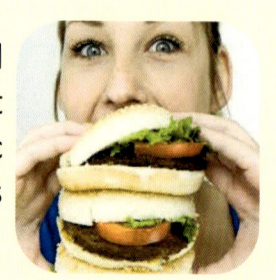

More weight and fat loss than low fat diets

Cutting carbs is one of the simplest and most effective ways to lose weight and body fat. Studies show that people having low carb high fat meals lose more weight, faster, than people on low-fat diets. Initially glycogen (carbohydrate storage) is reduced, this process also releases water. Excess water is also excreted from the body when insulin levels fall. Sodium is also lost in this process and it is important to consume adequate salt whilst the body is adapting to a very low carb lifestyle (see the salt section in "Essential tips to ensure success" on page 32).

The science supporting a very low carb/high fat lifestyle

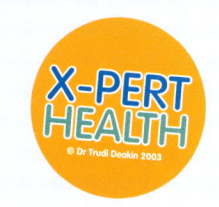

Once the body has adapted to the lifestyle, it becomes efficient at burning body fat instead of storing it. Lower levels of glucose and insulin mean that the switch to convert carbohydrate into fat is turned off and the fat burning switch is turned on. Fat then becomes the preferred fuel for energy which is good news as the body stores much more energy as fat than carbohydrate in everyone no matter what size or shape they are. Using fat stores for energy often leads to increased energy without the dips (daytime sleepiness or lethargy) that often accompanies high carbohydrate intake.

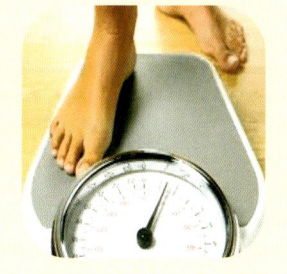

Another benefit shown in clinical studies is that the very low carb/high fat lifestyle is very effective at reducing the harmful abdominal fat that causes insulin resistance and increases the risk of Type 2 diabetes and heart disease.

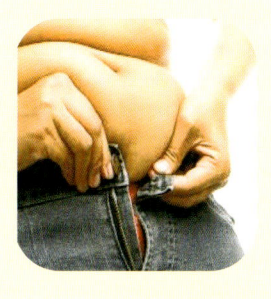

Blood glucose will reduce

Carbohydrate is the only nutrient that directly increases blood glucose levels. The amount of carbs you eat is the single most important factor for good blood glucose control. Once the amount of carbohydrate has been addressed, further improvements to blood glucose can be achieved by swapping carbs that release their glucose quickly (high glycaemic index "GI" foods) for slow releasing carb foods (low GI foods). Clinical trials have shown that people at risk of diabetes or with established diabetes can dramatically reduce their blood glucose levels so that they fall back into the normal healthy range. Prescribed diabetes medication is often significantly reduced and some people if they continue with the very low carb/high fat lifestyle may go into diabetes remission.

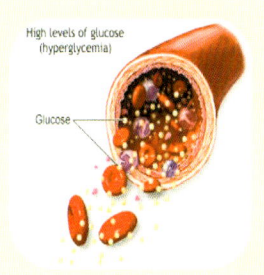

Blood pressure will reduce

High blood pressure is one of the strongest known risk factors for stroke and heart disease. Lowering blood pressure is therefore considered a very important step to lower the risk of cardiovascular disease. Studies indicate that adopting a low carb/high fat lifestyle may help people to lower blood pressure.

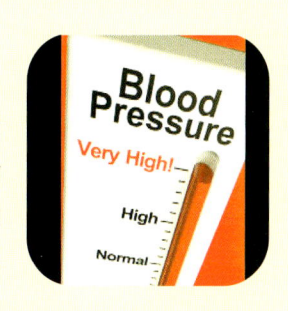

Triglyceride levels will reduce

Triglycerides are fat molecules. The main driver of increased levels of triglycerides in the blood is when carbs have been converted to fat rather than used for energy. It is well known that fasting triglycerides i.e. how much we have of them in the blood after an overnight fast, are a strong risk factor for heart disease and Type 2 diabetes. When people cut carbs, they tend to have a very dramatic reduction in blood triglycerides. In comparison, low-fat diets often result in an increase in blood triglycerides.

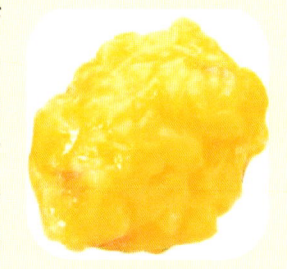

High Density Lipoprotein (HDL) will increase

HDL are like "road sweepers" mopping up as much excess cholesterol as possible and carrying it to the liver where it can be reused or excreted. HDL also stops the LDL particles from becoming damaged (oxidised) and causing fatty plaques. The higher your levels of HDL, the lower your risk of heart disease will be. One of the best ways to increase HDL levels is to eat fat - and low-carb meals include a lot of fat! Therefore, it is not surprising to see that HDL levels increase dramatically when adopting a low carb high fat dietary approach.

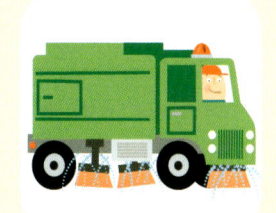

www.xperthealth.org.uk

The science supporting a very low carb/high fat lifestyle

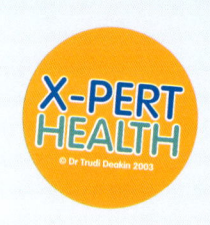

Reduction of small dense LDL and the number of LDL particles.
Low Density Lipoprotein (LDL) is often called the "bad" cholesterol. However, it is not the cholesterol that is the problem, cholesterol is essential to life! We need it for making body cells, hormones and for food digestion. It is the particles in the blood, the lipoproteins, that carry the cholesterol that can be a problem to health. LDL particles exist in different sizes, small dense "cars" and large fluffy "trucks". Many recent studies have looked into the importance of LDL particle number and size. The research has shown that people whose LDL particles are predominantly small and dense have a threefold greater risk of coronary heart disease because they easily mix with oxygen and slither into inflamed areas on the blood vessel wall forming fatty plaques. Furthermore, the large and fluffy type may actually be protective. Studies indicate carbohydrate restriction positively affects particle size by reducing the number of very small dense LDL particles (see pages 46-49). In the UK, LDL particle number and size is not routinely measured.

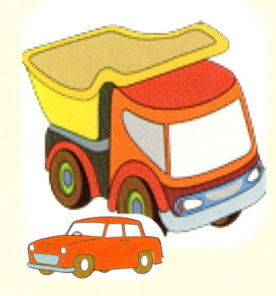

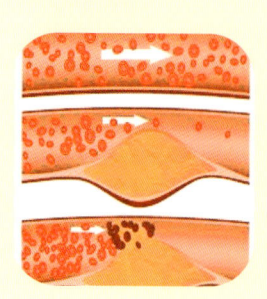

Insulin resistance will reduce and insulin levels will drop
Insulin clears glucose from the blood by opening the door into the body cells. Insulin resistance has become a very common problem leading to raised blood glucose levels and high levels of circulating insulin. Because insulin is a weight-promoting hormone, high levels encourage the storage of fat and it is also a risk factor for Type 2 diabetes and heart disease. Studies indicate that repeated exposure to insulin causes insulin resistance and carbohydrate restriction significantly lowers insulin levels compared to a low fat diet.

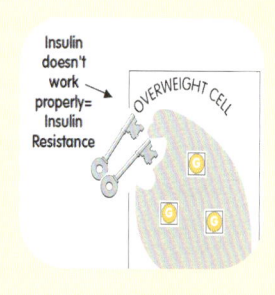

A reduction in prescribed medication
If you have diabetes and are on medication it is likely that you will be able to significantly reduce your prescribed medication because cutting carbs lowers blood glucose considerably. In one study, 95% of people with Type 2 diabetes managed to reduce or eliminate their glucose-lowering medication within 6 months. People who require insulin may be able to reduce their insulin requirement by 50%. However, due to the risk of low blood glucose (hypoglycaemia) it is important to discuss the very low carb/high fat lifestyle with your healthcare team before you start so that medication can be reduced.

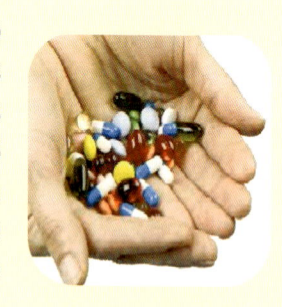

A reduced risk score for cardiovascular disease (CVD) - heart disease & strokes
The latest guidance from the National Institute for Health and Clinical Excellence (NICE) states that people older than 40 should have their CVD risk reviewed on an ongoing basis. Some risk factors such as age, sex, ethnicity and family history cannot be modified but others such as weight, blood pressure, LDL particle size and number can and restricting carbohydrate has been shown to reduce risk (see Health Indicators section pages 79 - 84).

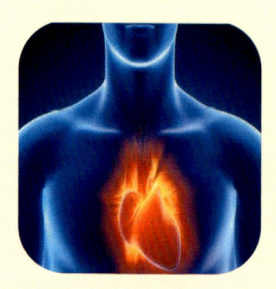

Improvement in liver function
The liver has many important functions which keep the body working normally. A healthy liver should contain little or no fat. However, 25-30% of people have the early form of non-alcoholic fatty liver disease (NAFLD). Carb restriction has been shown to reduce liver damage and the amount of fat stored in the liver. Adopting a low carb high fat dietary approach has shown a reduction in gamma-glutamyl transpeptidase (GGT), a marker for liver damage.

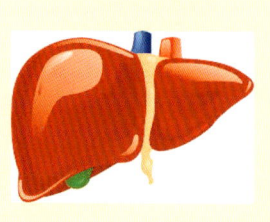

The science supporting a very low carb/high fat lifestyle

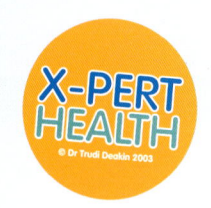

C-reactive protein (CRP) will be reduced
CRP can be measured in blood and is a known marker of inflammation and a risk factor for many conditions such as heart disease and Type 2 diabetes. Spikes in blood glucose and insulin resistance and consuming polyunsaturated fat* have all been shown to increase chronic (long-term) inflammation. There is evidence that the very low carb/high fat lifestyle not only prevents inflammation but also lowers blood levels of CRP and therefore reduces inflammation [*see section on dietary fats on pages 45 - 49].

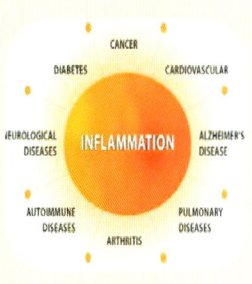

Improvements in acne and skin appearance
This lifestyle has been shown to be an effective treatment for spots and acne. This is partly due to the reduced inflammation (discussed above) and insulin resistance. Insulin stimulates the production of sebum (oil) in the skin. If this oil becomes oxidised it leads to pimples forming. Reduced insulin levels have been shown to lead to an improved complexion.

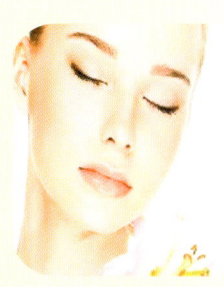

Reduced irritable bowel syndrome (IBS) symptoms
IBS is one of the most common gastrointestinal disorders seen worldwide, affecting up to 20% of the population of Western countries. One of its most frequent and bothersome symptoms is bloating and other symptoms include pain, diarrhoea and constipation. Research has shown that reducing carbs provides adequate relief, reduces abdominal pain, improves stool habits and quality of life in people suffering from IBS.

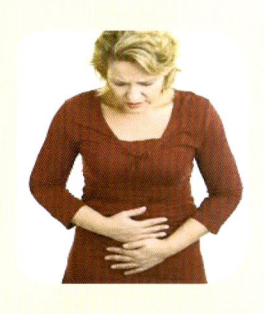

Improvements in heartburn and acid reflux
Heartburn and acid reflux symptoms are common complaints encountered in up to 40% of adults at some point in their lives. Heartburn is defined as a burning sensation whereas acid reflux is the regurgitation of stomach contents into the oesophagus. Clinical studies have reported that some individuals experienced complete and nearly immediate resolution of symptoms with this approach.

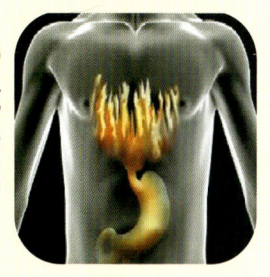

Improvements in polycystic ovarian syndrome (PCOS)
PCOS is a common condition affecting millions of women. Tiny cysts develop in the ovaries and affect the way the ovaries work. Symptoms of PCOS include irregular periods, increased body hair, being overweight, having acne, insulin resistance and fertility problems. There is no cure for PCOS but a very low carb/high fat lifestyle has been shown to significantly improve the symptoms.

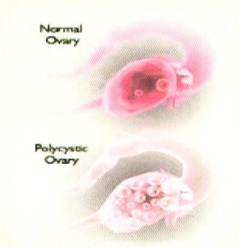

A reduction in premenstrual tension (PMT) symptoms
PMT is believed to affect approximately 80% women at some point in their lives. Some women are mildly affected, experiencing few symptoms, whilst for others PMT may seriously affect their lives on a monthly basis. The term PMT is used to describe a wide range of symptoms that occur after the middle of the menstrual cycle (ovulation) and disappear almost as soon as the period arrives. These symptoms can range from bloating, breast tenderness, migraines, depression, mood swings and food cravings. It has been shown that inflammatory factors may be elevated in women experiencing PMT and therefore the very low carb/high fat lifestyle may help to alleviate symptoms.

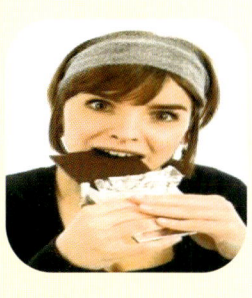

www.xperthealth.org.uk

The science supporting a very low carb/high fat lifestyle

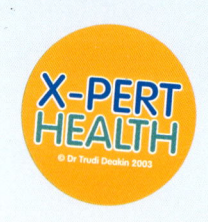

A reduction in oxidative stress and aging

The ketone arising from the very low carb/high fat lifestyle have been shown to slow the aging process in several ways: reducing oxidative damage within the body by producing antioxidants that stabilise toxic free radicals; reducing blood glucose and triglyceride levels which reduce the formation of advanced glycation end products (AGEs) that are linked to aging; reducing hunger and calorie consumption which decreases oxidative damage within the body. All these factors increase longevity and wellbeing.

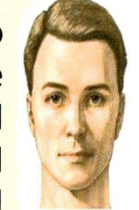

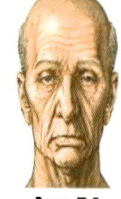

A possible treatment for neurological and neurodegenerative diseases

This dietary approach is well known in the epilepsy treatment field and is currently experiencing a revival as a treatment for epileptic seizures, especially in children. The diet is extremely effective and more importantly, it's non-toxic and well tolerated.

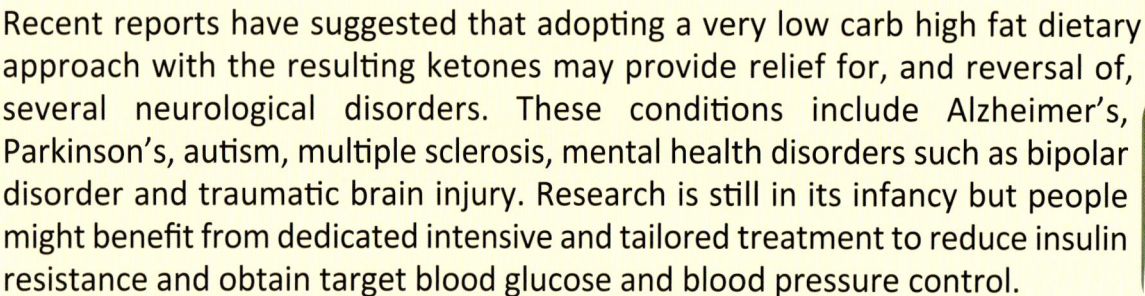

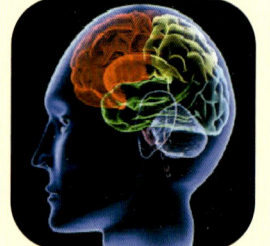

Recent reports have suggested that adopting a very low carb high fat dietary approach with the resulting ketones may provide relief for, and reversal of, several neurological disorders. These conditions include Alzheimer's, Parkinson's, autism, multiple sclerosis, mental health disorders such as bipolar disorder and traumatic brain injury. Research is still in its infancy but people might benefit from dedicated intensive and tailored treatment to reduce insulin resistance and obtain target blood glucose and blood pressure control.

A possible treatment for cancer

It has been suggested that a low carb high fat lifestyle may help to control cancer. Most cancer cells thrive exclusively on glucose. Normal cells can use either glucose or ketones for fuel. The growth of cancer cells may be suppressed by 1) consuming very few carbs and 2) lowered insulin levels. When glucose is lowered via the diet, normal cells can switch to burning ketones for fuel and survive quite nicely, while the cancer cells are starved of the glucose they need to grow. Work is in the early stages and much more research is needed. The advantage of this treatment is that it is non-toxic to the rest of the body.

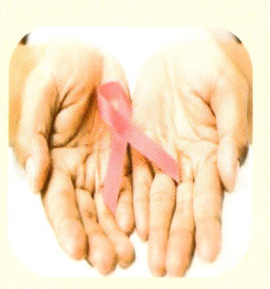

How could this lifestyle benefit me?

Low carb high fat dietary approaches have been controversial for decades demonised by fat-phobic health professionals and the media who were in support of the low fat/high carb diet. It was believed that a high fat intake would raise cholesterol and cause heart disease.

However... times are changing. In the past decade hundreds of studies have been conducted on low carb diets. In almost every study, carbohydrate restriction was shown to be more beneficial than the traditional low fat diet. These clinical trials have failed to report any negative findings and have in fact reported improvements in many of the conditions such as blood cholesterol levels.

If you experience any of the conditions listed above, you may wish to try this approach to see if it works for you. If this is the case, read on....

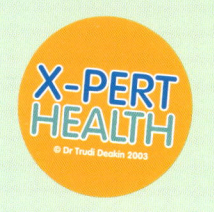

This dietary approach is not a quick fix

Changing the way you live your life is never easy! We are creatures of habit. This means that we prefer to keep the status quo and do things the way we have always done them. Changing our ways can often make us feel awkward and uncomfortable. Therefore, we are unlikely to change our lifestyle unless we think it is really going to be worth it and we are going to reap the benefits.

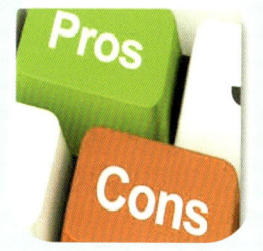

Diets are frequently broken when the burden outweighs the benefit i.e. people start craving foods that they have omitted. Yo-yo dieting generally leads to weight gain and poorer health outcomes. To prevent this it is better to think about changing your lifestyle on a permanent basis and making changes that you will be happy with maintaining during the rest of your life.

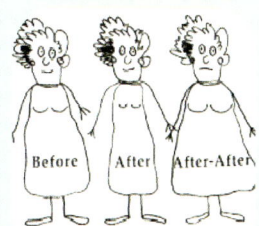

The low carb dietary approach appears to be particularly effective for up to 6 months, but if people revert to their old ways, the benefits will not be sustainable i.e. the weight will creep back up. It is much more appropriate to think of low-carb as a lifestyle, NOT a diet. The only way to succeed in the long-term is to stick to it. The top tip for doing this to ensure that you satisfy your palate on a daily basis. This means making sure that you enjoy what you eat.

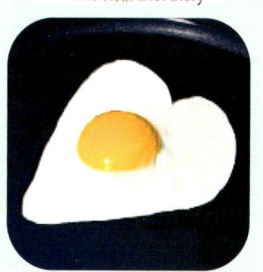

Questions to ask yourself before starting

1. What do I hope to achieve from adopting a very low carb/high fat dietary approach?
....
....

2. How will I know if it is working for me?
....
....

3. What will I find easy?
....
....

4. What will I find difficult?
....
....

5. What could I do to get extra support?
....
....

6. How could I remove some of the barriers?
....
....

7. When would be a good time to start?
....
....

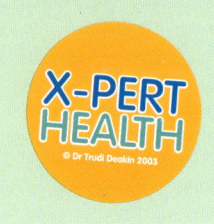

Step 1: What are you currently eating?

Instructions

Before you start you need to determine the sources and amount of carbohydrate in your current diet. There are two food diaries overleaf. Complete one food diary with what you eat on a typical weekday (page 11) and the remaining food diary with the food eaten on a weekend day (page 12).

Examples of food are as follows:

Starches: cereal, bread, potato, rice, pasta, chapatti, naan, couscous

Vegetables: carrots, broccoli, cauliflower, sweetcorn, peas, courgette, peppers, mushrooms, salad

Fruit: apple, orange, banana, grapes, berries (strawberry, raspberry, blueberries, red currant) nectarine, plums, dried fruit, tomato

Milk & Dairy: milk, yogurt, cheese (state whether full fat, semi-skimmed, skimmed, low fat)

Protein: meat, fish, eggs, pulses, nuts

Fats/Sweets: oil, spreads, butter, mayonnaise, cream, chocolate, desserts, sweets

Ready Meal or Takeaway: lasagne or Indian meal (state the food manufacturer if possible)

Beverages: coffee/tea (state whether you have milk and sugar), fruit juice, fizzy drinks, alcoholic drinks

Comments: state how the food product has been cooked, for example, in breadcrumbs, in oil, in a tomato-based, cream or cheese sauce, gravy, steamed etc.

Top tip: Sometimes it is difficult to remember exactly what you have eaten at the end of the day so it may help you to complete the diary as you go through the day.

Example of completed food diary for breakfast and mid-morning snack

Food Group	Food Name and Amount (house measure e.g. tablespoon or weight)
Breakfast	
Starches	Cornflakes (6 tablespoons), toast (wholemeal) x 2 slices
Vegetables	None
Fruits	Blueberries added to cereal (1 tablespoon)
Milk & Dairy	Milk (semi-skimmed) added to cereal (200ml)
Protein	Boiled egg (x1)
Fats/Sweets	Margarine (x2 teaspoons) on toast, raspberry jam x 1 teaspoon
Ready Meal or Takeaway	None
Beverages	Orange juice (150ml), coffee with semi-skimmed milk and x1 teaspoon sugar
Comments	Bread toasted / egg boiled / salt added to egg
Snack	
	2 x Coffee with semi-skimmed milk and x1 teaspoon sugar
	2 x Rich Tea biscuits

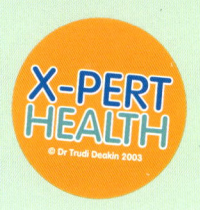

Step 1: What are you currently eating? Weekday

Food Group	Food Name and Amount (house measure e.g. tablespoon or weight)
Breakfast	
Starches	
Vegetables	
Fruits	
Milk & Dairy	
Protein	
Fats/Sweets	
Ready Meal or Takeaway	
Beverages	
Comments	
Snack	
Lunch	
Starches	
Vegetables	
Fruits	
Milk & Dairy	
Protein	
Fats/Sweets	
Ready Meal or Takeaway	
Beverages	
Comments	
Snack	
Dinner	
Starches	
Vegetables	
Fruits	
Milk & Dairy	
Protein	
Fats/Sweets	
Ready Meal or Takeaway	
Beverages	
Comments	
Snack	

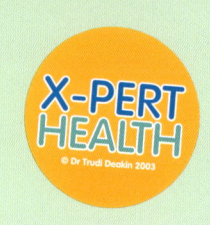

Step 1: What are you currently eating? Weekend

Food Group	Food Name and Amount (house measure e.g. tablespoon or weight)
Breakfast	
Starches	
Vegetables	
Fruits	
Milk & Dairy	
Protein	
Fats/Sweets	
Ready Meal or Takeaway	
Beverages	
Comments	
Snack	
Lunch	
Starches	
Vegetables	
Fruits	
Milk & Dairy	
Protein	
Fats/Sweets	
Ready Meal or Takeaway	
Beverages	
Comments	
Snack	
Dinner	
Starches	
Vegetables	
Fruits	
Milk & Dairy	
Protein	
Fats/Sweets	
Ready Meal or Takeaway	
Beverages	
Comments	
Snack	

Step 2: Identification of carbohydrate food

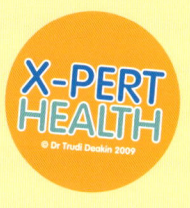

Instructions

Once you have identified what carbohydrate food you are currently eating you can replace it with non-carbohydrate food sources such as fat. With a pen, highlight or ring the foods that contain carbohydrate. Use the following sections in the handbook to help you:

1) Sources of carbohydrate - page 14
2) Carbohydrate content of everyday foods - pages 58 to 68
3) Foods that contain none or a little (green light), moderate (amber light) or high (red light) amounts of carbohydrate - page 15 to 17
4) Alcohol - pages 50 to 51

Example of identifying carbohydrate foods

Food Group	Food Name and Amount (house measure e.g. tablespoon or weight)
Lunch	
Starches	*Baked potato - 200g (cooked)*
Vegetables	Salad - lettuce (handful), tomato (x1), cucumber (3cm chunk)
Fruits	*Banana x 1 (medium-sized)*
Milk & Dairy	Grated cheese (30g)
Protein	*Baked beans (x1 small tin)*
Fats/Sweets	Mayonnaise (low fat) x 1 dessert spoon
Ready Meal or Takeaway	None
Beverages	1 can Diet Coke
Comments	Potato cooked in the microwave
Snack	
3pm	*1 x yogurt (Muller light strawberry)*
	2 x coffee *(semi-skimmed milk with x 1 sugar)*
Dinner	
Starches	*Pasta spirals - white (250g cooked or 5 tablespoons)*
Vegetables	Sweetcorn x 1 tablespoon, broccoli x 1 tablespoon
Fruits	*Tomato (chopped x ½ tin 200g)*
Milk & Dairy	None
Protein	Chicken fillet (150g uncooked)
Fats/Sweets	Vegetable oil x 1 tablespoon, *2 scoops of vanilla ice cream*
Ready Meal or Takeaway	None
Beverages	Red wine - 175ml (medium glass)
Comments	Chicken & tomato pasta sauce made in frying pan using vegetable oil
Snack	
9pm	*Orange (medium-sized)*
10pm	*Hot chocolate drink (low fat)*

Please note: salad ingredients, vegetables and the red wine have not been highlighted because they only contain small amounts of carbohydrate. However, if eaten/drunk to excess or consumed in a concentrated form e.g. chopped tomatoes, they may add sufficient carbs that need to be counted.

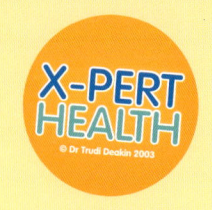

Step 2: Identification of carbohydrate food

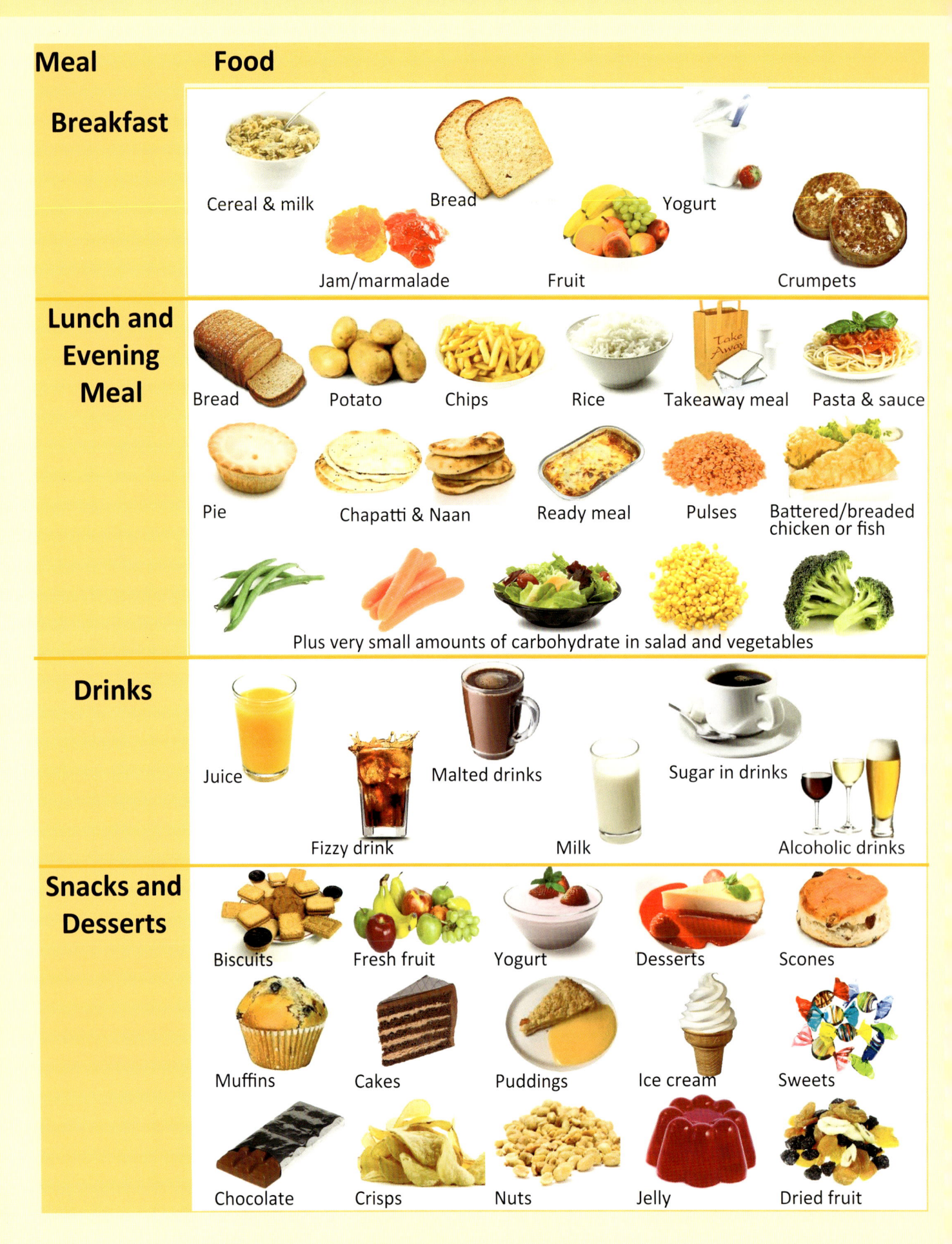

Meal	Food
Breakfast	Cereal & milk, Bread, Yogurt, Crumpets, Jam/marmalade, Fruit
Lunch and Evening Meal	Bread, Potato, Chips, Rice, Takeaway meal, Pasta & sauce, Pie, Chapatti & Naan, Ready meal, Pulses, Battered/breaded chicken or fish. Plus very small amounts of carbohydrate in salad and vegetables
Drinks	Juice, Fizzy drink, Malted drinks, Milk, Sugar in drinks, Alcoholic drinks
Snacks and Desserts	Biscuits, Fresh fruit, Yogurt, Desserts, Scones, Muffins, Cakes, Puddings, Ice cream, Sweets, Chocolate, Crisps, Nuts, Jelly, Dried fruit

www.xperthealth.org.uk

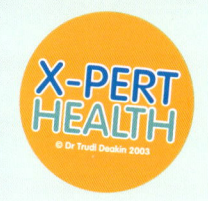

Step 3: Eliminating carbs - how low do you go?

A very low carb/high fat lifestyle provides just 20 to 50g of carbs per day.
At this level of carbohydrate restriction, the brain and central nervous system cannot obtain the 130g of glucose per day that it requires and therefore fat stores are broken down to produce a chemical called ketones. Ketones can supply the essential energy required for the brain and this reduces dependency on dietary carbohydrate. Blood levels of glucose and insulin drop enabling the body to start burning fat. If you omit all the carbohydrate sources that you have highlighted in your food diary in Step 2, then it is likely that you are consuming less than 50g carbs per day.

Foods high in carbohydrate to eliminate (red light)
These foods contain more than 10g carbs per portion and should normally be omitted to reduce carbs to between 20g and 50g per day. You may occasionally have a small portion for a treat.

Starches:
All breakfast cereals, bread (including gluten free), baps, finger roll, baguette, bagel, muffin, crumpet, fruit tea cake, potato (boiled, baked, mash, chips, French fries), rice, pasta, ravioli, noodles (egg & rice), vermicelli, gnocchi, chapatti, naan, paratha, puri, roti, brioche, croissant, pain au chocolat, couscous, crackers & crispbread, croutons, ciabatta, panini, focaccia, pitta bread, flatbread, tortilla, poppadom, pancakes, waffle, hot cross bun, scones, rice cakes, dumplings, Yorkshire pudding, stuffing, hash brown, potato croquette, eba/gari, yam, bulgur wheat, quinoa, polenta

Vegetables:
Sweet potato, butternut squash, parsnips, plantain, sweetcorn, beetroot, onion rings

Fruit:
Apple, orange, banana, grapes, nectarine, plums, cherries, dried fruit (dates, figs, prunes, raisins, sultanas), tinned fruit, grapes, mango, melon, persimmon, peach, pear, pineapple, banana chips

Milk & Dairy:
Yogurt with added sugar and fruit, custard, milk pudding, milkshake

Protein:
Pulses - mushy peas, baked beans, butter & kidney beans, chickpeas, lentils. Meat, poultry or fish coated in batter or breadcrumbs (e.g. chicken kiev, fish fingers, battered fish, scampi, calamari), Scotch egg, savoury pies & sausage rolls, haggis, seafood sticks, cashew & soya nuts

Fats/Sweets:
All desserts & puddings, sweet pies, biscuits, cakes, sweets, chocolate, confectionery, fancy ice cream, sorbet, jelly, mousse, crisps, Bombay mix, popcorn, pretzels, tortilla chips, prawn crackers, jam, marmalade, honey, syrup, lemon curd, chocolate spread, sugar, chutney, tomato, brown & chilli sauce

Ready Meal or Takeaway:
Any meals that include pasta, potato, rice, chapatti, naan such as lasagne, cottage pie, Chinese chow mein, sweet & sour, pizza, bhaji, spring roll, samosa, pakora, burgers

Beverages:
Sugar added to coffee/tea, cappuccino, latte, hot chocolate, all fruit juices, smoothie, sugar-sweetened cordial & fizzy drinks. Alcohol - sweet wines & liqueurs, cider, alcopops, ale & carb-rich lager & beer (see alcohol section on pages 50 to 51)

Step 4: What can you eat?

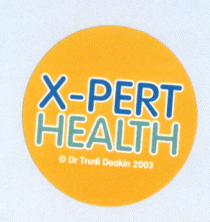

Food to be eaten in moderation (amber light)

These foods contain small amounts of carbohydrate (2g to 10g per serving) and therefore if eaten to excess, it could result in the total carbohydrate for the day being greater than 50g.

The carbohydrate content of common foods are listed on pages 58 to 68 and this may help you determine your portion size.

Starches:
Coconut flour, soya flour (ground almonds can also be used as a flour substitute)

Vegetables:
Peas, bean sprouts, brussel sprouts, carrots, mangetout, onion, coleslaw, soup (fresh, tinned or homemade without starch filler), gherkins, pickled onion

Fruit:
Berries (such as strawberries, raspberries, blueberries, blackberries, black/redcurrants), apricot, clementine, satsuma, fig, kiwi, papaya or plum. Pomegranate, half grapefruit, rhubarb (no added sugar), tomato (fresh, tinned, sun-dried)

Milk & Dairy:
Full fat milk, full fat natural yogurt, coconut milk, unsweetened soya milk, raita

Protein:
Black pudding, sausages, pâté, BBQ ribs. Whole nuts (almonds, brazil, hazelnuts, macadamia, peanuts, pecan, pistachio, walnuts, pine nuts), ground almonds, seeds, Marmite, peanut butter, houmous, Quorn

Fats/Sweets:
Desserts, puddings, cakes & biscuits made with flour substitutes and artifical sweetener (see recipe section), Greater than 70% cocoa chocolate, no-added sugar chocolate, gravy made with granules, sauce (horseradish, mint, roux, piccalilli, soy, tartare, Worcestershire), salad cream, full fat salad dressing, single, whipping, clotted, soured & double cream, creme fraiche

Ready Meal or Takeaway:
Meat, fish, vegetable-based with no rice, pasta, potato or bread. The following may be sufficiently low carb: Indian curries *without* rice, chapatti or naan; Chinese stir-fry *without* rice or noodles; kebabs with salad and without the pitta bread and sushi containing a small amount of rice.

Beverages:
Milk in coffee/tea, dry white wine, red wine, champagne, some brands of beer/lager (see alcohol section on pages 50 to 51)

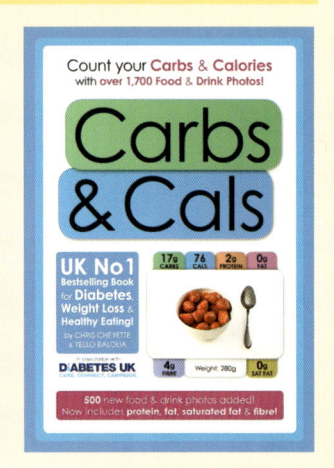

Another method to assess the amount of carbohydrate you are eating is to use the Carbs & Cals book or mobile phone app, which can be used as a visual carbohydrate and calorie counter. For more information visit: http://www.carbsandcals.com/

The book/app contains around 1,700 food and drink photos, with the carbohydrate, calorie, protein, fat and fibre content clearly displayed in colour-coded tabs around each photo. There are up to 6 portion photos for each food item, which allows you to identify your portion size and easily assess the carbs. There are 26 different colour-coded sections that enable you to make informed choices about the carbohydrate you eat.

Step 4: What can you eat?

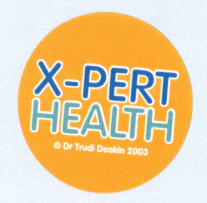

Food containing virtually no carbohydrate (green light)

These foods contain very few carbs and should be eaten to satisfy the appetite. **It is very important to eat sufficient fat**. Trying to remain on a low fat diet whilst also cutting carbs fails to satisfy the appetite. The key to success is to embrace dietary fat and use it to satisfy the palate so you are less likely to crave carbohydrate or snack between meals. Information about the type of dietary fat to consume can be found on pages 45 - 49.

Starches:

Starches are rich in carbohydrate so many need omitting (see red light box on page 15). Any flour substitute such as ground almonds, golden milled flaxseed, coconut flour or soya flour can be eaten in moderation (see amber light box on page 16)

Vegetables:

Asparagus, aubergine, avocado, bamboo shoots, broad beans, broccoli, cabbage, cauliflower, celery, courgette, cucumber, edamame beans, green beans, leeks, lettuce, mushrooms, okra, pak choi, peppers, rocket, spinach, spring greens, turnip, watercress, olives, guacamole

Fruit:

All fruit contains some carbohydrate and therefore needs to be avoided (see red light box on page 15) or portion controlled (see amber light box on page 16)

Milk & Dairy:

Cheese - all types and varieties except those with added fruit such as apricots and cranberries

Protein:

All meat, poultry, fish & seafood

Processed meat - high meat content (98%) sausage & beef burgers, chorizo, pancetta, parma ham, prosciutto, salami, pork scratching, luncheon meat

Eggs (boiled, scrambled, fried, poached, omelette), tofu

Fats/Sweets:

Olive, coconut & palm oil, butter, lard, mayonnaise (full fat), cream, artificial sweeteners, gravy made with meat juices, sauces (bearnaise, hollandaise, cream), mustard, pesto

Ready Meal or Takeaway:

Meat or fish sashimi

Beverages:

Black coffee or tea, artificially-sweetened cordial and sugar-free fizzy drinks

N.B. Alcoholic drinks - spirits such as vodka, gin, rum & whiskey do not contain carbohydrate but need to be mixed with sugar-free drinks and consumed within government recommendations (see alcohol section on pages 50 to 51)

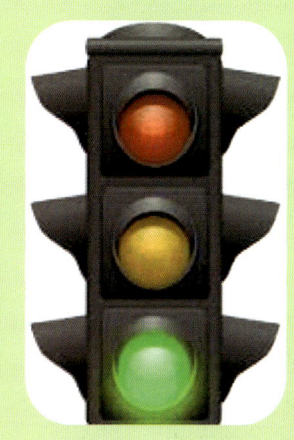

Step 4: What can you eat?

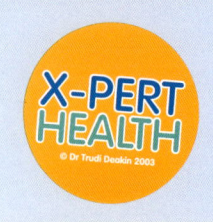

The success of a very low carb/high fat lifestyle depends on the amount of carbohydrate restriction, the level of fat substitution and the length of time you remain on the diet. As discussed previously, it should not be seen as a quick fix but a long-term approach to healthy living. Planning is key. It will help if you know what foods you are going to replace your favourite carb staples with.

The list below may provide some ideas for swaps:

Breakfast - replace cereal and toast with:
- different varieties of cooked breakfast (eggs, bacon, high meat content (98%) sausages, mushrooms & tomato fried in butter)
- berries with full fat Greek yogurt
- walnut scone (see recipe) with butter

Lunch - replace a sandwich, wrap or baked potato with:
- chicken/meat with salad or vegetables
- smoked/tinned/fresh fish with salad or vegetables
- omelette with cheese/mushrooms or tomato
- low carb bread (see recipe for English muffin)

Evening meal - meat or fish but replace potato, rice, pasta, chapatti or naan with:
- cauliflower mash (see recipe)
- carrot, swede or celeraic fries (see recipe)
- courgette spaghetti (see recipe)
- stir-fry (meat, fish or vegetable)
- lasagne with leek pasta (see recipe)
- vegetables or salad
- frittata (an egg-based dish similar to an omelette or crustless quiche, enriched with additional ingredients such as meats, cheeses, vegetables - see recipe)

Desserts/cakes/biscuits - see recipes

Snacks
- low carb tree nuts (walnuts, Bazil nuts, almonds)
- pork scratchings
- berries with double cream

The *recipe section* can be located on pages 72 to 77

Overleaf a traditional low fat/high carbohydrate diet is compared with a low carb/high fat diet that contains 36g of carbohydrate. This may provide you with ideas on how to change your diet. You may further reduce your carb intake to nearer 20g per day by having less milk in drinks or using cream instead. **Suggested meal plans** can be located on pages 69 & 70.

Top tip: as the very low carb/high fat lifestyle increases satiety (the feeling of fullness) many people experience a reduced appetite and report that they only require two meals each day rather than three meals and snacks. This is fine unless you take medication that needs to be taken with food throughout the day. If this is the case you will need to arrange a medication review with your healthcare team.

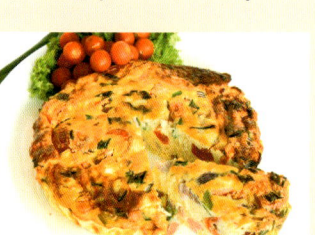

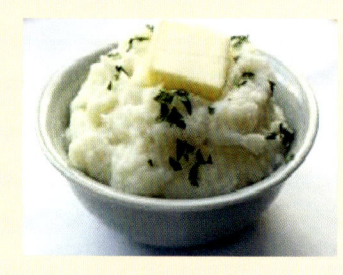

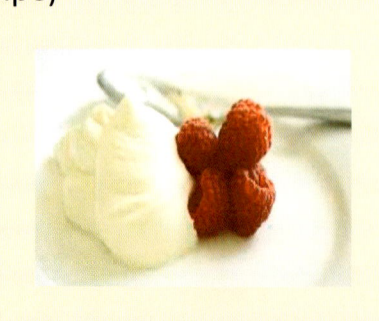

Step 4: What can you eat?

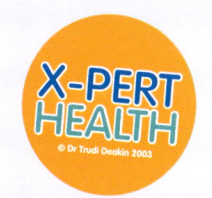

Comparison of dietary approaches

Low fat/high carb	Kcal	Fat (g)	Carbs (g)	Very low carb/high fat	Kcal	Fat (g)	Carbs (g)
Breakfast				**Breakfast**			
Fruit & Fibre (4 tbs/30g)	140	2	28	Fried egg x 1	90	7	0
Semi-skimmed milk (125 ml)	60	2	6	Grilled bacon x 2 rashers (36g)	168	14	0
Granary bread (1 slice/40g)	95	1	18	Grilled tomato (80g)	14	0	3
Jam (1 tsp/15g)	40	-	10	Fried mushrooms in butter (40g)	63	7	0
Pure orange juice (200 ml)	86	-	18	Coffee/tea (milk added for day)	0	0	0
Snack				**Snack**			
Piece of fruit (80g)	46	-	18				
Lunch				**Lunch**			
Carrot/butter bean soup ½ tin	117	4	17	Mackerel fillet (75g)	266	23	0
Pitta bread (x1)	190	1	38	Lettuce (80g)	10	0	2
Salad (tomato/lettuce)	20	-	4	Tomato x1 large (130g)	22	0	4
Salmon (tinned, 50g)	75	4	-	Cucumber (5cm/80g)	8	0	1
Reduced fat mayo (1 tsp/5g)	30	3	1	Mayonnaise full fat x 1 tbs (15g)	104	11	0
Low fat yogurt (200g pot)	106	0	17	Almonds (30g)	185	16	2
Snack				**Snack**			
Reduced fat crisps (1 pk/30g)	132	6	16				
Evening Meal				**Evening Meal**			
Pork loin (100g)	129	2	-	Roast chicken quarter (150g)	209	9	0
4 x new potato (200g)	152	0	37	Broccoli (80g)	19	1	1
Carrots (80g)	19	0	4	Carrots (80g)	19	0	4
Broccoli (80g)	19	1	1	Gravy from meat juices (50ml)	99	10	2
Bisto (50 ml)	14	1	2	Sugar-free jelly (1 pot 140ml)	8	0	0
Banana (100g)	79	0	19	Whipped cream (30 ml)	112	12	1
Low fat ice-cream (1 scoop)	80	2	15	Strawberries x 5 (80g)	22	0	5
Supper				**Supper**			
Options drink	40	1	6	Glass of red wine (175ml)	119	0	1
Chocolate (4 squares/20g)	115	8	9	Cheese (50g)	208	18	0
Milk in 5 coffee/teas Semi-skimmed milk (200ml)	98	3	10	**Milk in 5 coffee/teas** Full fat milk (200ml)	130	7	10
TOTAL (g) **Percentage (%)**	1882 Kcal	41g 20%	294g 62%	**TOTAL** **Percentage (%)**	1875 Kcal	135g 65%	36g 8%

Kcal = calories, Carbs = carbohydrate, tsp = teaspoon, tbs = tablespoon

Please Note: This information was correct at the time of printing but different brands may have a different nutritional content.

Step 5: Monitoring success

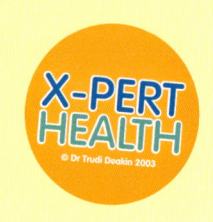

There are 5 food groups: fruit & vegetables; proteins; fats; milk & dairy; carbohydrates. For decades people have been advised to have fewer portions of fat and more portions of carbs. The very low carb/high fat dietary approach encourages 5-14 portions of fat and just 0-2 portions of carbohydrate per day. The sample low carb day on page 19 has been plotted on the Nutrition for Health template below using the "What is a portion" resource on page 21.

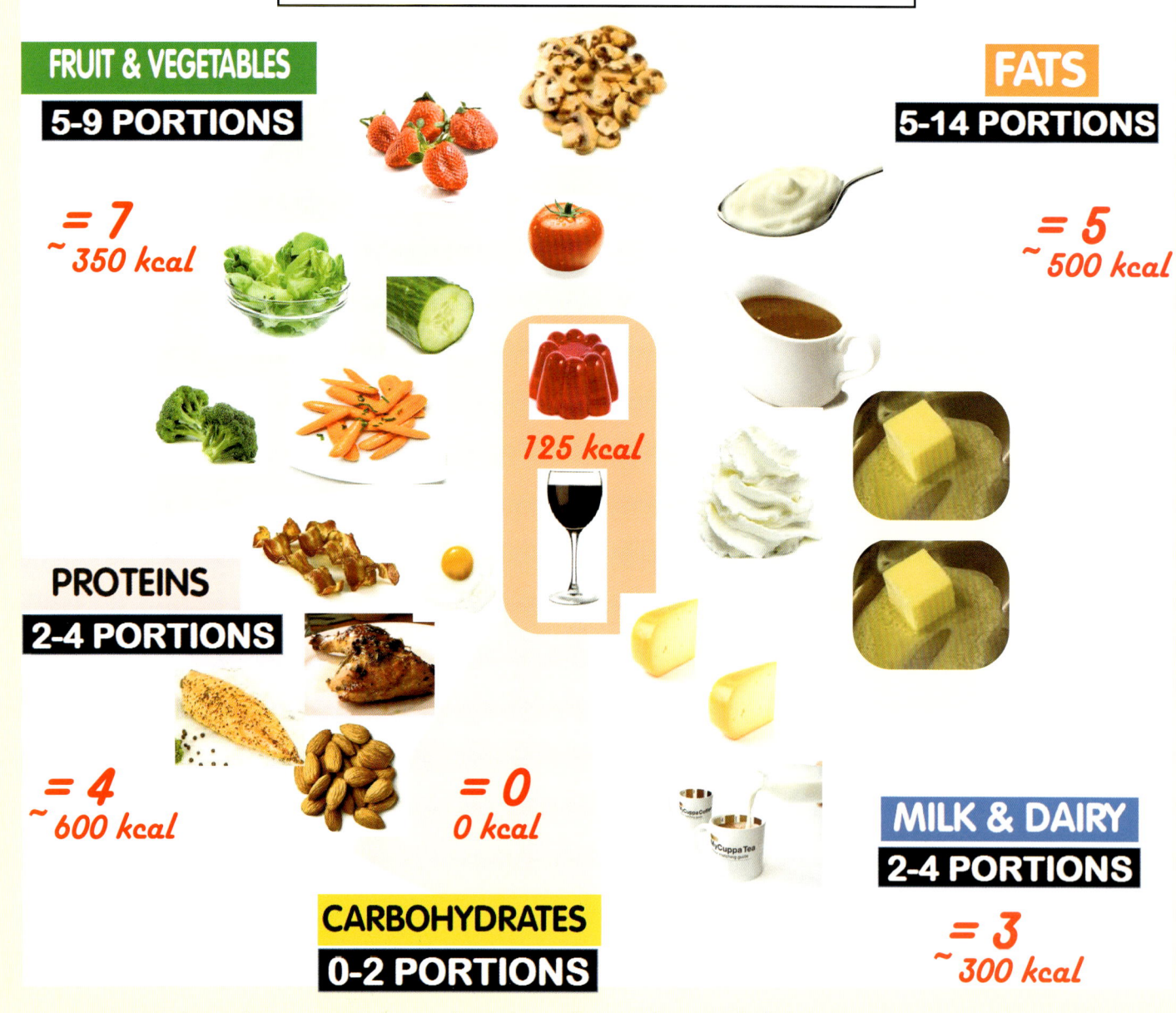

Nutrition for Health

FRUIT & VEGETABLES
5-9 PORTIONS
= 7
~ 350 kcal

FATS
5-14 PORTIONS
= 5
~ 500 kcal

125 kcal

PROTEINS
2-4 PORTIONS
= 4
~ 600 kcal

= 0
0 kcal

MILK & DAIRY
2-4 PORTIONS
= 3
~ 300 kcal

CARBOHYDRATES
0-2 PORTIONS

Assumptions have been made regarding the calories that each food group contributes to the total energy intake. The sample diet therefore contains:

- Fat — 5 portions — 500 calories
- Fruit & Vegetables — 7 portions — 350 calories
- Proteins — 4 portions — 600 calories
- Milk & Dairy — 3 portions — 300 calories
- Carbohydrates — 0 portions — 0 calories
- Alcohol & low calorie sweetener — 2 portions — 125 calories
- **TOTAL** — **1875 calories**

Step 5: Monitoring success

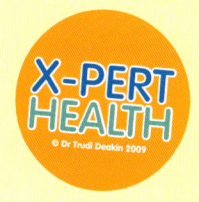

FOOD GROUP	DAILY PORTIONS	WHAT IS A PORTION?
Fats (contain monounsaturated, saturated & polyunsaturated fatty acids) **100 kcal/portion**	**5 to 14 portions** Avoid processed polyunsaturated vegetable oils such as corn, sunflower, soybean, canola, cottonseed, safflower	○ 1 heaped tsp butter (13g) ○ 1 level tsp lard or ghee (10g) ○ 1 tbs oil (12g) ○ 1 tbs full fat mayonnaise (15g) ○ 4 tbs single cream (50g) ○ 2 tbs double cream (20g) ○ 2 tbs creme fraiche (30g) ○ 4 tbs meat juice gravy (100g)
Fruit & Vegetables (contains fibre, vitamins and minerals) **50 kcal/portion**	**5 to 9 portions** (80g per portion) Include a mixture of vegetables, salad and fruit daily - at least 400g per day [fresh, frozen, tinned]	○ 2-3 tbs low carb vegetables (80g) ○ Side salad (80g) ○ 1 medium tomato or 4 cherry tomatoes ○ 1-2 tbs berries (80g) ○ 3 tbs stewed rhubarb with artificial sweetener (80g) ○ Olives (50g) ○ ¼ avocado (40g)
Meat, Fish, Poultry & Alternatives (contains protein) **150 kcal/portion**	**2 to 4 portions** oily fish: 2 portions per week for girls & pre-menopausal women, up to 4 portions per week for post-menopausal women, men and boys Try to have grass-fed cattle & free-range eggs	○ 80-100g red meat, chicken or oily fish ○ 120-140g white fish (unbattered) ○ 2 eggs ○ 2-3 rashers bacon (45g) ○ 2 thin or 1 thick sausage (50g) (98% meat) ○ 3 slices salami/8 slices chorizo (40g) ○ 2 tbs nuts/peanut butter (25g) ○ 1 tbs ground almonds (25g)
Milk & Dairy Food (contains calcium) **100 kcal/portion**	**2 to 4 portions** Choose full fat and try different varieties of cheese	○ ⅓ pint (200ml) full fat milk ○ 2-3 tbs full fat Greek/natural yogurt (100g) ○ Cheese - matchbox-size chunk (35g) ○ 60 ml coconut milk ○ ⅔ pint (400ml) unsweetened soya milk ○ 6 tbs raita (seasoned indian yogurt) (100g)
Carbohydrate **80 kcal/portion**	**0 to 2 portions** Low carb flour substitutes	○ 1 tbs coconut flour (25g) ○ 1 tbs soya flour (25g)
Drinks zero calories (milk counted in milk section)	Drink plenty - aim for at least 6 - 8 cups/mugs/glasses per day [2 litres]	○ 1 mug coffee/tea (200-250ml) ○ 'No added sugar' squash/fizzy drink ○ Water
Alcoholic Drinks **100k cal/portion**	Up to 2-3 units a day for women Up to 3-4 units a day for men	2 units of alcohol is: ○ 1 pint beer/lager/cider (4%) ○ 1 medium glass (175ml) of wine ○ 1 double pub measure of spirits
Zero and low calorie sweeteners	Zero or low calorie sweeteners in place of sugar can be used in drinks, yogurt, fruit and in baked products	○ zero calories = 1 tsp stevia, Canderel, Splenda, Sweetex, erythritol ○ low calorie = 1 tsp xylitol (2 calories)

Please note: 1 tsp = 1 teaspoon, 1 tbs = 1 tablespoon

www.xperthealth.org.uk

Step 5: Monitoring success

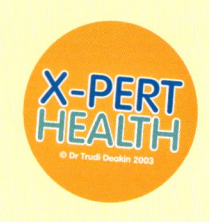

Assess your diet to see if you are successfully adopting the very low carb/high fat lifestyle

This is a simple tool that enables you to assess your dietary intake very quickly. You can plot your daily intake of food and drink and it provides you with immediate feedback informing you if you are managing to replace your carb intake with dietary fat.

To complete the dietary self-assessment follow these steps:

1. Plot what you eat or drink throughout the day (this is easier than trying to remember what you have eaten later on) on the Nutrition for Health template (opposite).

2. For each food/drink ask yourself: "which food group does it belong in?" and "how many portions does my serving contain?" For guidance refer to 'What is a portion?' on the previous page.

3. Add up the number of portions from each food group.

4. If you wish, you can also estimate total daily calories intake by adding-up the number of calories consumed from each food group. This is only an estimation but you can see that when the sample daily intake on page 19 has been plotted onto the Nutrition for Health template on page 20, the total calories for the day remain the same whether calculated or estimated. Therefore if you do want to keep a check on your daily calories, this is a simple and useful tool to use.

5. A sample low carb daily intake has been completed on page 24 to provide further guidance.

6. Please email admin@xperthealth.org.uk to obtain a copy of the Nutrition for Health template that you will be able to print and use as frequently as you wish.

- 1 portion (P) of **fats** is 100 Kcal
- 1 portion (P) of **fruit/vegetables** is 50 Kcal
- 1 portion (P) of **milk & dairy** is 100 Kcal;
- 1 portion (P) of **protein foods** is 150 Kcal;
- 1 portion (P) of **starchy carbohydrate** is 80 Kcal
- 1 unit (U) of **alcohol** is 100 Kcal

Questions to ask yourself about your daily intake

- Am I having **sufficient portions of fat** (between 5 and 14 portions)? Am I choosing monounsaturated & saturated fats in preference to processed polyunsaturated oils?
- Am I eating between **5 and 9 portions of fruit & vegetables**? Am I choosing low carbohydrate varieties?
- Am I having **2 to 4 portions of milk and dairy food**? Am I choosing the full fat options?
- Am I having **2 to 4 portions of protein foods**? Am I choosing a variety of white/oily fish, meat, eggs & nuts (tofu or quorn if vegetarian)? Am I able to source grass-fed cattle?
- Have I managed to omit **starchy carbohydrates** and only use flour substitutes in moderation (up to 2 portions)? Am I having enough fibre from other sources?
- How many **units of alcohol** am I having? Am I sticking to 2-3 units (female) or 3-4 units (male)?

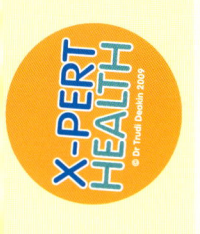

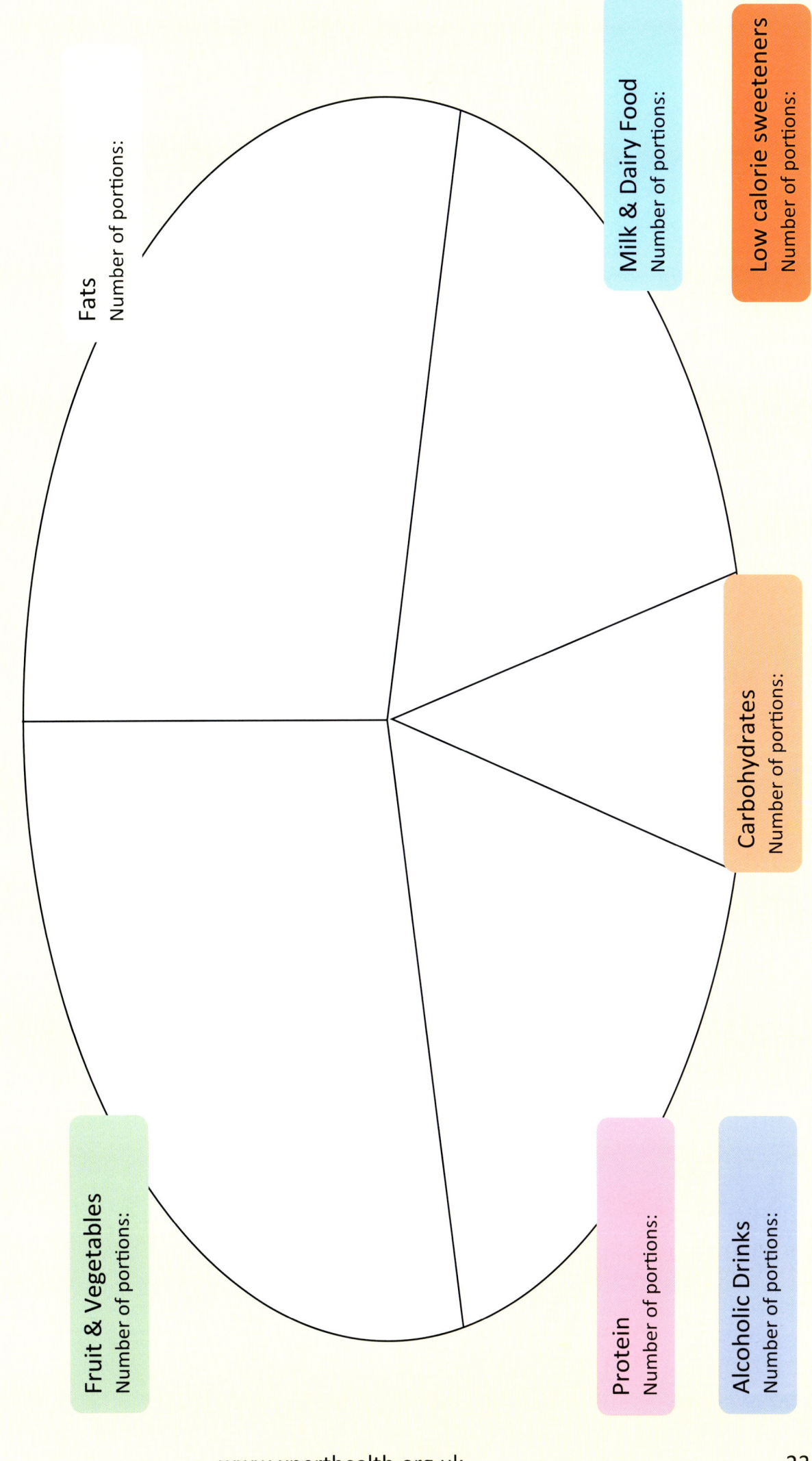

Step 5: Monitoring success

Fats
Number of portions:

Milk & Dairy Food
Number of portions:

Low calorie sweeteners
Number of portions:

Carbohydrates
Number of portions:

Fruit & Vegetables
Number of portions:

Protein
Number of portions:

Alcoholic Drinks
Number of portions:

www.xperthealth.org.uk

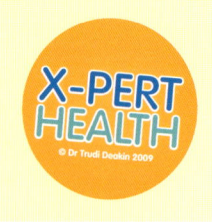

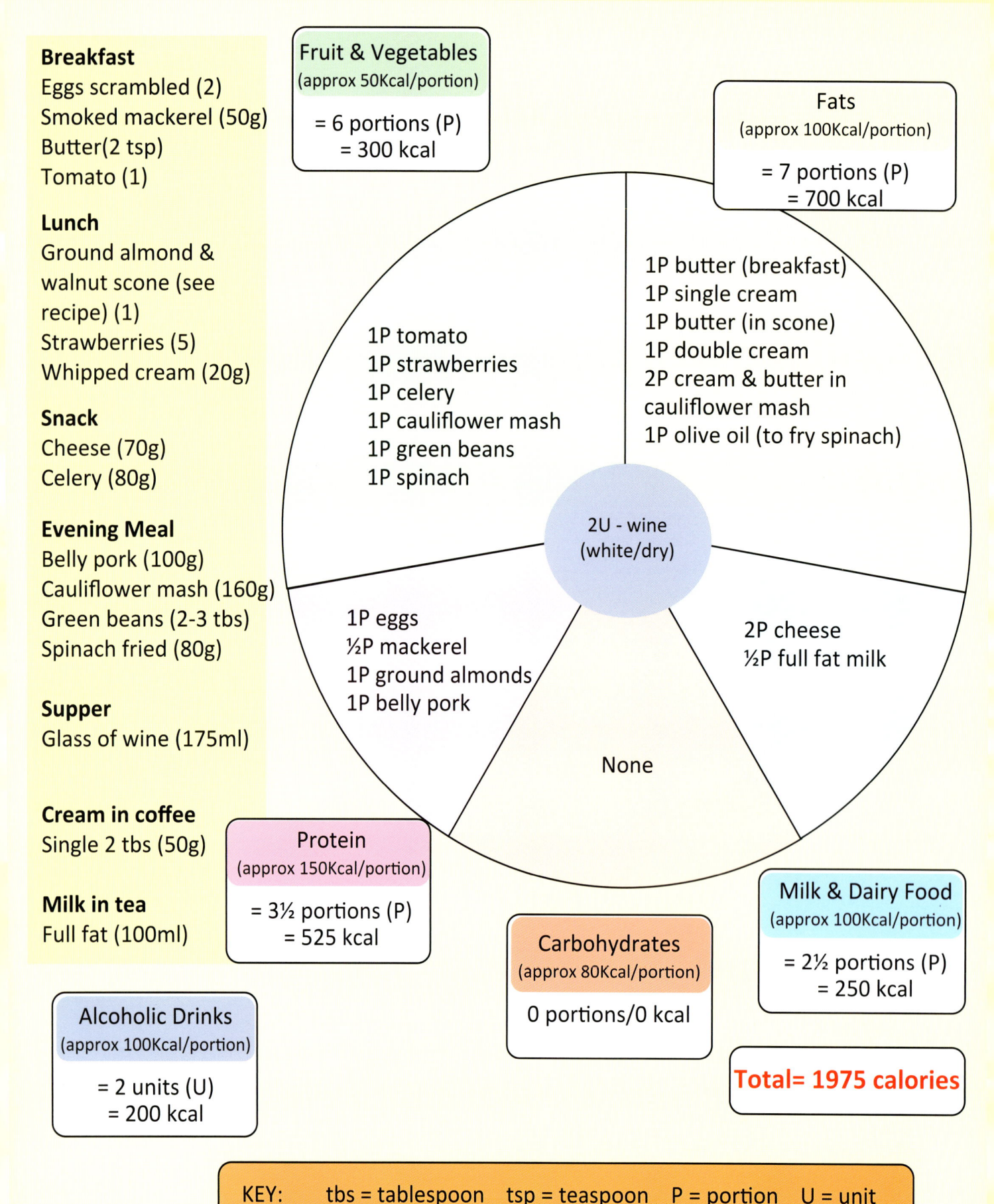

Step 5: Monitoring success

Breakfast
Eggs scrambled (2)
Smoked mackerel (50g)
Butter (2 tsp)
Tomato (1)

Lunch
Ground almond & walnut scone (see recipe) (1)
Strawberries (5)
Whipped cream (20g)

Snack
Cheese (70g)
Celery (80g)

Evening Meal
Belly pork (100g)
Cauliflower mash (160g)
Green beans (2-3 tbs)
Spinach fried (80g)

Supper
Glass of wine (175ml)

Cream in coffee
Single 2 tbs (50g)

Milk in tea
Full fat (100ml)

Fruit & Vegetables
(approx 50Kcal/portion)
= 6 portions (P)
= 300 kcal

- 1P tomato
- 1P strawberries
- 1P celery
- 1P cauliflower mash
- 1P green beans
- 1P spinach

Fats
(approx 100Kcal/portion)
= 7 portions (P)
= 700 kcal

- 1P butter (breakfast)
- 1P single cream
- 1P butter (in scone)
- 1P double cream
- 2P cream & butter in cauliflower mash
- 1P olive oil (to fry spinach)

Protein
(approx 150Kcal/portion)
= 3½ portions (P)
= 525 kcal

- 1P eggs
- ½P mackerel
- 1P ground almonds
- 1P belly pork

Milk & Dairy Food
(approx 100Kcal/portion)
= 2½ portions (P)
= 250 kcal

- 2P cheese
- ½P full fat milk

Carbohydrates
(approx 80Kcal/portion)
0 portions / 0 kcal

None

Alcoholic Drinks
(approx 100Kcal/portion)
= 2 units (U)
= 200 kcal

2U - wine (white/dry)

Total = 1975 calories

KEY: tbs = tablespoon tsp = teaspoon P = portion U = unit

Step 5: Monitoring success

Another method of monitoring success is by using tools available on the internet or via mobile phone apps.

One example is "My Fitness Pal" that you can access either via the internet (http://www.myfitnesspal.com) or via an app (iPhone App Store or Google Play). Although this programme advertises itself as a calorie tracker, it also enables you to obtain a breakdown of calories consumed from fat, protein and carbohydrate.

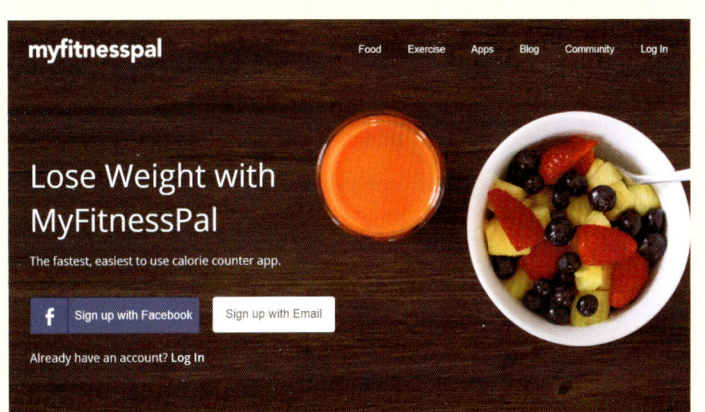

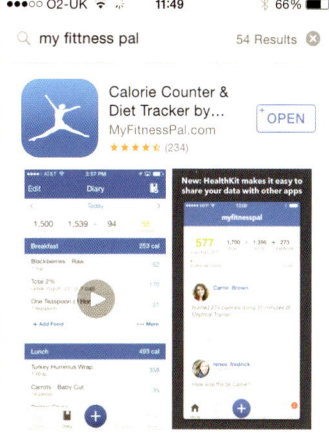

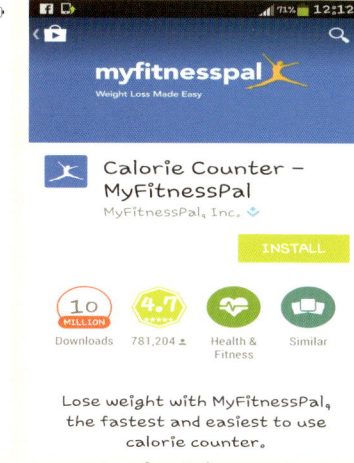

Internet version　　　　　　　　　**iPhone version**　　　　　　　**Android version**

Instructions

1. Create a profile. This will involve you providing a username, email address and password.
2. You will be asked to enter your current weight, height, goal weight, sex and date of birth in addition to activity levels. These answers are used to calculate your energy (calorie) requirements.

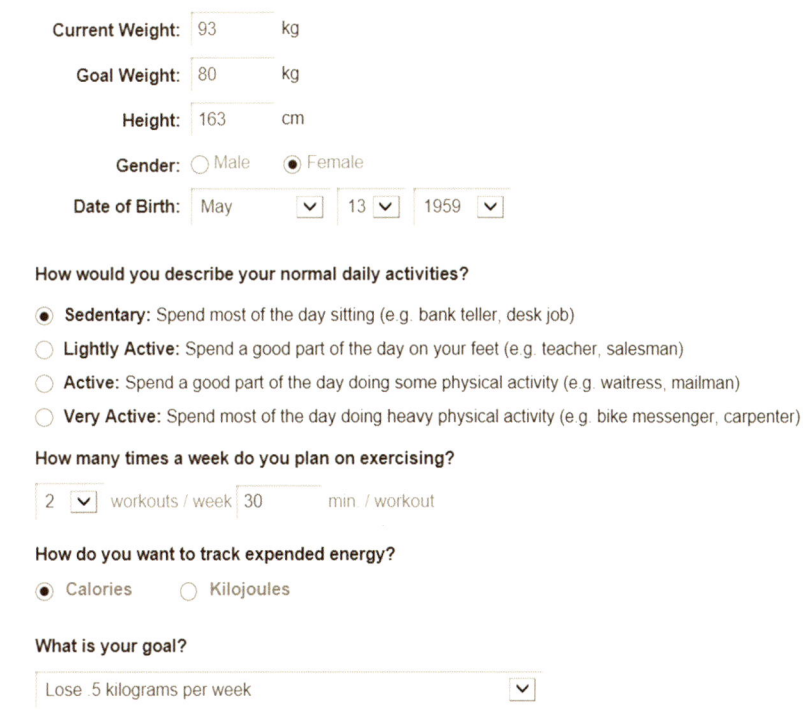

Current Weight: 93 kg
Goal Weight: 80 kg
Height: 163 cm
Gender: ○ Male ● Female
Date of Birth: May 13 1959

How would you describe your normal daily activities?
- **Sedentary:** Spend most of the day sitting (e.g. bank teller, desk job)
- **Lightly Active:** Spend a good part of the day on your feet (e.g. teacher, salesman)
- **Active:** Spend a good part of the day doing some physical activity (e.g. waitress, mailman)
- **Very Active:** Spend most of the day doing heavy physical activity (e.g. bike messenger, carpenter)

How many times a week do you plan on exercising?
2 workouts / week   30 min. / workout

How do you want to track expended energy?
● Calories ○ Kilojoules

What is your goal?
Lose 5 kilograms per week

Where it states "What is your goal?" If you wish to reduce or increase your weight it is realistic to aim for 0.5 to 1kg(1 or 2 lbs) per week.

Step 5: Monitoring success

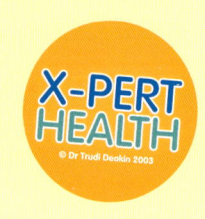

3. The system will automatically generate calorie, fat, protein and carb recommendations for you but **BE AWARE** because these will be based on a low fat/high carbohydrate dietary plan until you change them!

Your Fitness Goals

Nutritional Goals	Goals
Net Calories Consumed* / Day	1,340 cal/day
Carbs / Day	168.0 g
Fat / Day	45.0 g
Protein / Day	67.0 g

Fitness Goals	Goals
Calories Burned / Week	450 cal/week
Workouts / Week	2 Workouts
Minutes / Workout	30 mins

Your Diet Profile	Target
Calories Burned	
From Normal Daily Activity	1,890 cal/day
Net Calories Consumed*	
Your Daily Goal	1,340 cal/day
Daily Calorie Deficit	550 calories
Projected Weight Loss	0.5 kg/week

* Net Calories Consumed = Total Calories Consumed - Exercise Calories Burned

[Change Goals]

4. Click onto the green box "**Change Goals**". At this point you will have an option of choosing *Guided* or *Custom* goals. Click onto "**Custom**" and then "**Continue**".

Change Your Fitness Goals

How would you like to change your fitness goals?

○ **Guided:** Update my profile and have MyFitnessPal determine my goals automatically **(Recommended)**

● **Custom:** Manually set my own custom fitness goals

[Continue]

Step 5: Monitoring success

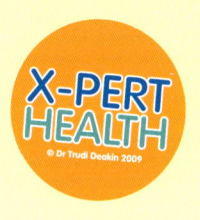

5. You are then able to change any of the goals. In the example below Mrs Bloggs has decided that she wishes to reduce her daily calories to 1500. To follow a very low carbohydrate diet she has identified that she would like 10% of her calories to be from carbohydrate, 60% from fat and 30% from protein. The new goals need to be entered and saved.

Daily Nutritional Goals	Targets
Net Calories Consumed*	1,500 calories
Carbohydrates	10% — 38.0g
Protein	30% — 113.0g
Fat	60% — 100.0g

To follow a very low carb/high fat lifestyle, the amount of carbohydrate consumed per day should be less than 50g. Some people decide to be very strict and set a 5% goal for carb intake (19g for a 1500 calorie diet). Protein intake is normally between 15-30% depending on total calorie intake and fat should provide the greatest proportion of calories at 60 to 70%.

6. You can now start to enter the food and drink you consume for each meal and snack. If you are using a mobile phone app, you will have an option to scan the barcode with your phone and this saves time in searching for the food products.

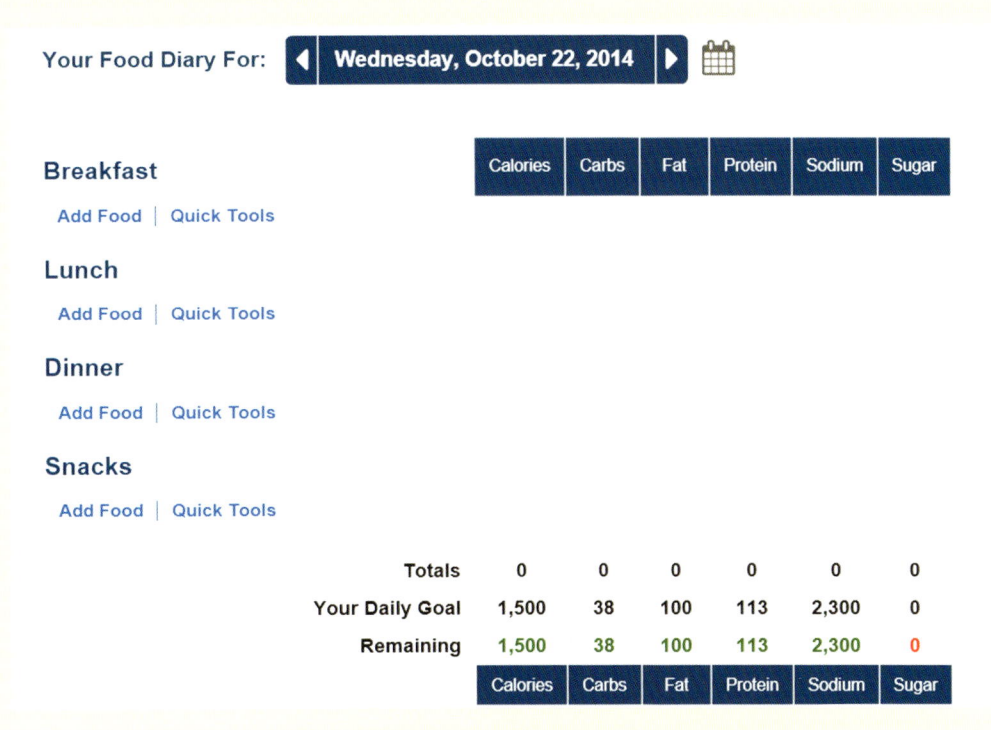

Your Food Diary For: Wednesday, October 22, 2014

	Calories	Carbs	Fat	Protein	Sodium	Sugar
Breakfast Add Food | Quick Tools						
Lunch Add Food | Quick Tools						
Dinner Add Food | Quick Tools						
Snacks Add Food | Quick Tools						
Totals	0	0	0	0	0	0
Your Daily Goal	1,500	38	100	113	2,300	0
Remaining	1,500	38	100	113	2,300	0
	Calories	Carbs	Fat	Protein	Sodium	Sugar

Please note: some food products have been entered by members of the public rather than food manufacturers and therefore may only provide an estimation rather than accurate information. Some food products will also have incomplete nutritional information.

Step 5: Monitoring success

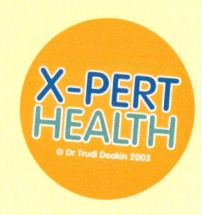

Option to search for a food/drink OR...

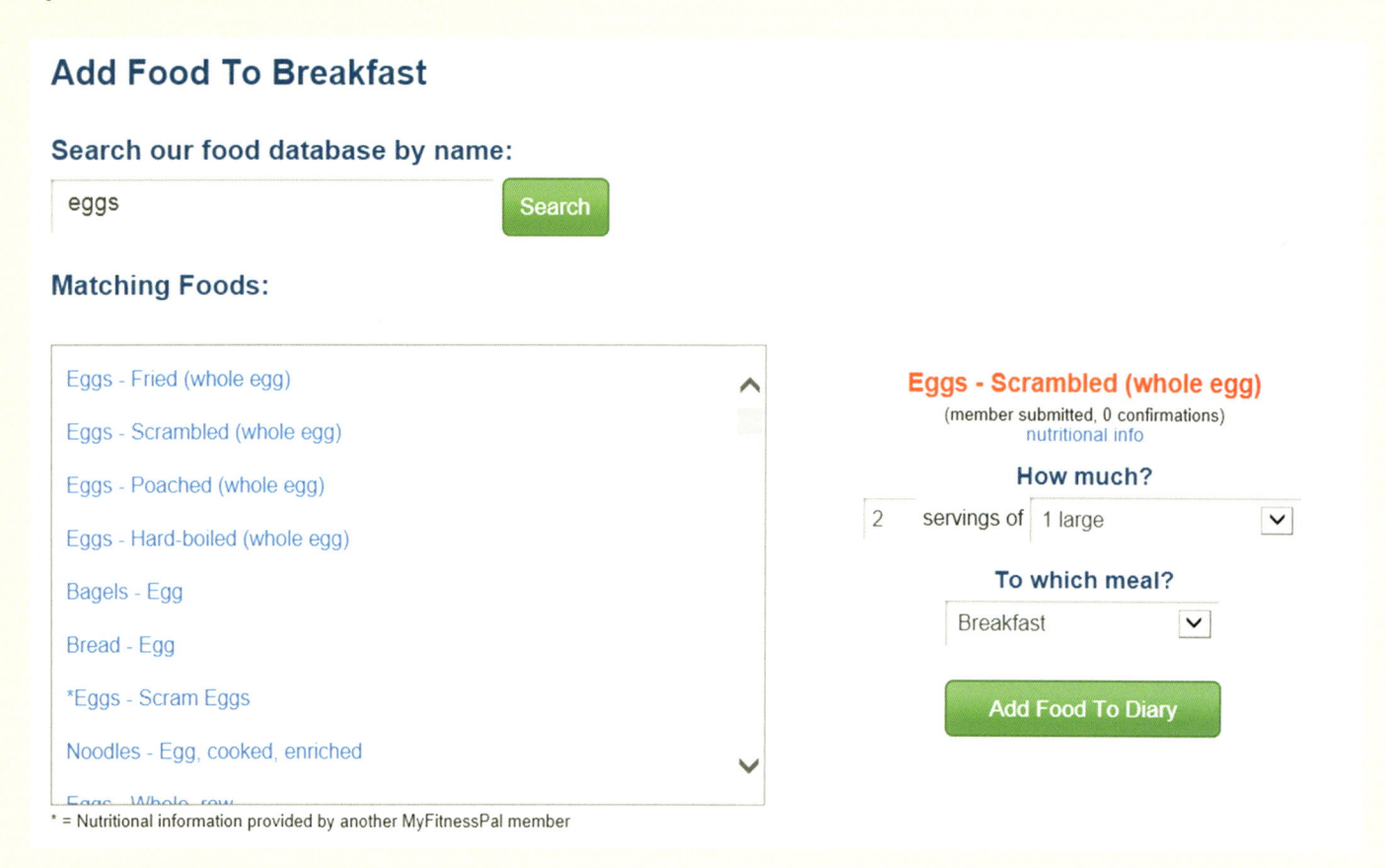

Add Food To Breakfast

Search our food database by name:

[eggs] [Search]

Matching Foods:

- Eggs - Fried (whole egg)
- Eggs - Scrambled (whole egg)
- Eggs - Poached (whole egg)
- Eggs - Hard-boiled (whole egg)
- Bagels - Egg
- Bread - Egg
- *Eggs - Scram Eggs
- Noodles - Egg, cooked, enriched
- Eggs - Whole, raw

* = Nutritional information provided by another MyFitnessPal member

Eggs - Scrambled (whole egg)
(member submitted, 0 confirmations)
nutritional info

How much?

2 servings of 1 large

To which meal?

Breakfast

[Add Food To Diary]

........Option to scan a barcode with a mobile phone but remember to check weight/portion size

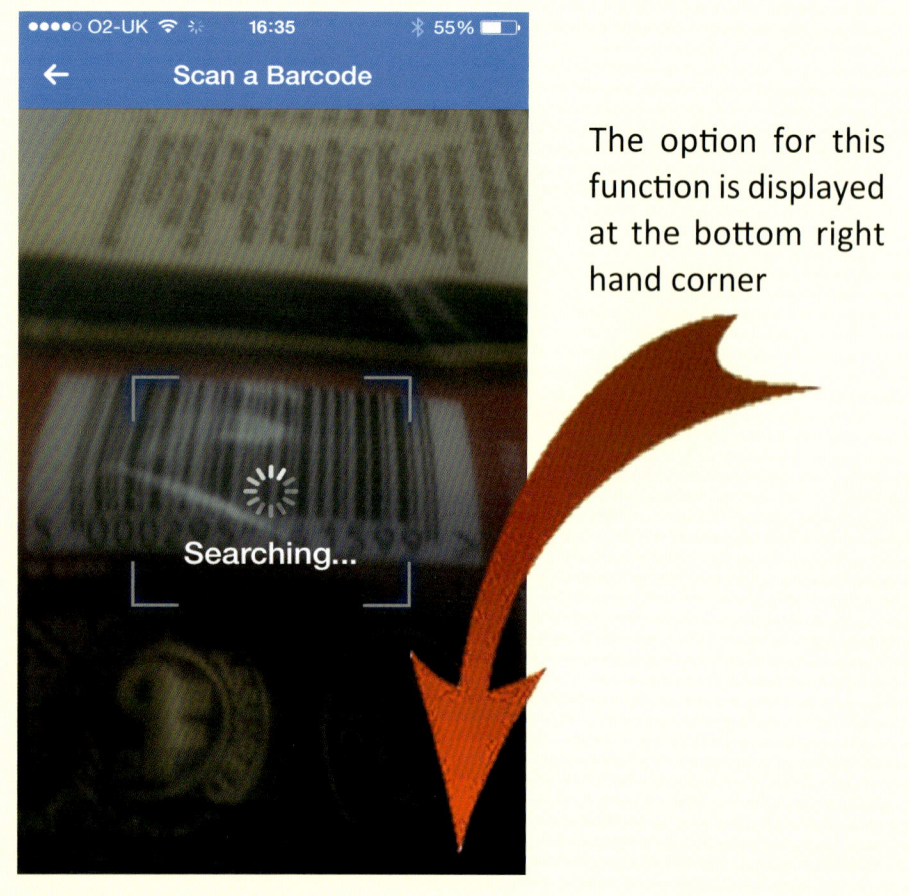

The option for this function is displayed at the bottom right hand corner

Step 5: Monitoring success

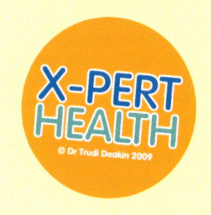

8. Once you have entered all the food and drink for the day it will summarise your dietary intake and compare it to your goals.

Breakfast	Calories	Carbs	Fat	Protein
Tesco - Smoked Mackerel Fillet 100g, 50 g	155	0	12	11
Butter - Salted, 26 g(s)	186	0	21	0
Tomato - Tomato, 1 whole, medium	15	3	0	1
Eggs - Scrambled (whole egg), 2 tbsp	45	1	3	3
Add Food | Quick Tools	401	4	36	15

Lunch				
Asda - Ground Almonds, 25 g	161	2	14	6
Butter - Salted, 26 g(s)	186	0	21	0
Sainsbury's - Double Cream, 20 ml	88	0	10	0
Strawberries - Raw, 5 small (1" dia)	11	3	0	0
Walnuts - Walnut Pieces, 0.1 oz (14 halves)	19	0	2	0
Add Food | Quick Tools	465	5	47	6

Dinner				
Cauliflower - Cooked, boiled, drained, with salt, 160 g	37	7	1	3
Asda - Green Beans, 80 g	22	4	0	1
Spinach - Sauteed Spinach, 1 cup cooked	41	7	1	5
Butter - Unsalted, 13 g(s)	93	0	11	0
Generic - Roasted Pork Belly, 100 grams (cooked weight)	293	0	21	25
Oil - Olive, 1 tsp	40	0	5	0
Add Food | Quick Tools	526	18	39	34

Snacks				
Cheddar - Cheddar, 80 g	322	1	27	20
Celery - Raw, 1 serving	15	3	0	1
Generic - Wine, White Dry 175ml, 175 ml	116	0	0	0
Generic - Milk Full Fat, 100 ml	64	5	4	3
Generic - Single Cream, 30 ml/2fl oz.	59	1	6	1
Add Food | Quick Tools	576	10	37	25

	Calories	Carbs	Fat	Protein
Totals	1,968	37	159	80
Your Daily Goal	1,500	38	100	113
Remaining	-468	1	-59	33

Step 5: Monitoring success

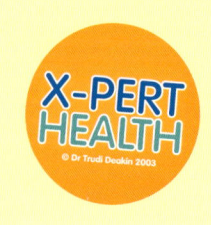

9. The day's food intake plotted on page 29 is the same diet that was plotted using the low carb Nutrition for Health template on page 24. Amazingly, although both tools only provide an estimation, the total calories for the day differ by only 7 calories.

10. If using the mobile phone application, clicking on *"more"* at the bottom right-hand corner will enable you to either obtain a nutritional breakdown for the day or a pie chart demonstrating the percentage breakdown from fat, protein and carbohydrate for a particular day or averaged over a week. The sample below would confirm that you are achieving your target of consuming less than 10% of calories from carbohydrate, between 60-80% from fat and 15-30% from protein.

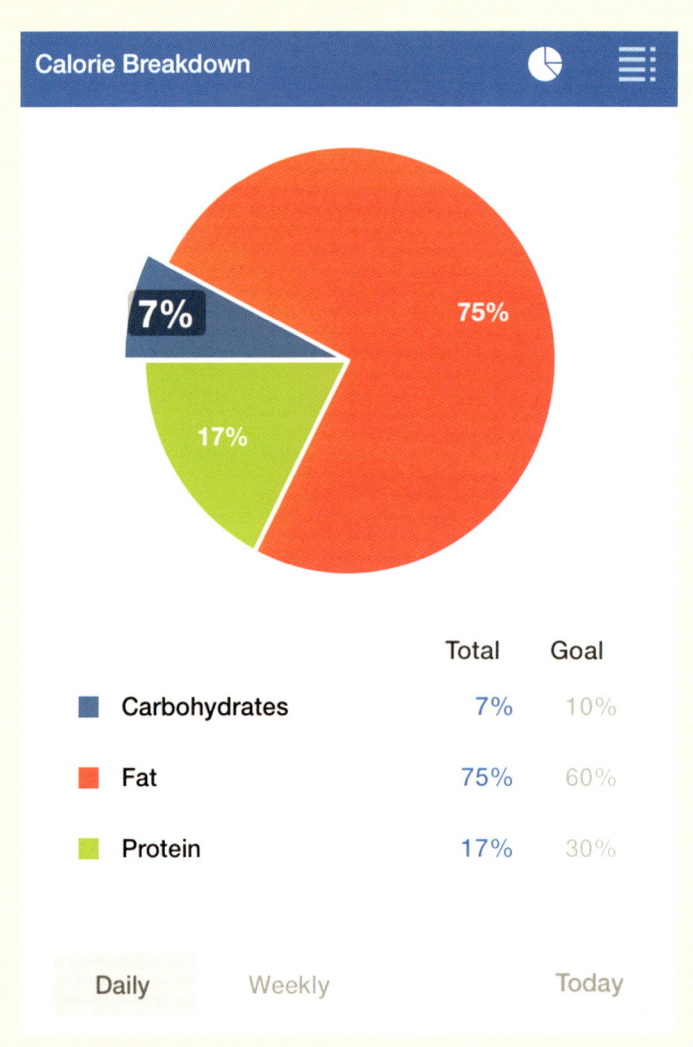

	Total	Goal
Carbohydrates	7%	10%
Fat	75%	60%
Protein	17%	30%

The final word on monitoring success

You may, or may not, wish to use the dietary tools to estimate the calorie and carb content of your very low carb/high fat lifestyle. However, it is recommended that you do keep a record of your weight and any symptom relief you may experience. At the back of the handbook (pages 85 to 89) there is a section to help you do this.

In addition, health results monitored by your healthcare team are explained with an opportunity to assess the impact of your new very low carb high fat lifestyle on these results over a period of time.

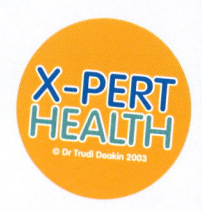

Step 6: Maintenance

Once you have achieved your desired goal, whether it is weight change, symptom relief, increased energy or all of these, you need to decide what you are going to do. There are three options:

1. Remain on a very low carb/high fat lifestyle

If you have experienced benefits from restricting carbohydrate and have satisfied your palate by ensuring that you have consumed sufficient dietary fat, you may be happy to remain on a diet consisting of 20g-50g of carbohydrate per day. It is possible to have a nutritionally complete intake with this dietary approach and clinical studies have not reported health problems from people remaining on this lifestyle long-term.

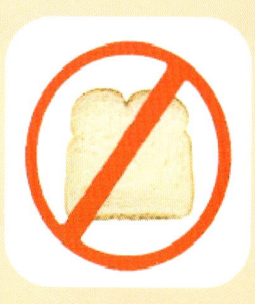

2. Gradually increase carbs to determine the level that retains the benefits (e.g. weight loss or symptom relief) but enables you to consume more carbohydrate

If you have struggled with the lifestyle and have missed consuming carbohydrate you may wish to experiment with gradually increasing carbs to see if you are able to maintain your weight or remain symptom free. You could try increasing carbohydrate by 10-20g each week but cut back if weight gain or symptoms return. A standard low carb diet is below 130g per day (see carbohydrate restriction definitions on page 2).

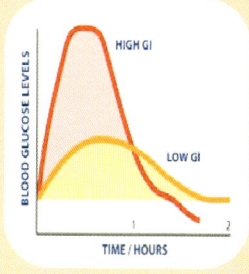

If you have benefited from the very low carb/high fat lifestyle then it is recommended that you remain on a relatively low carb diet by not increasing your daily carbohydrate intake to above 130g and choosing slow releasing (low glycaemic index "GI") carbs (see GI section on page 55).

Another thing to consider is the reason why you decided to try a very low carb/high fat lifestyle in the first place. Some of the benefits are due to the production of ketones and carbohydrate intake does have to be very low (usually less than 50g per day) for the body to make ketones. Ketones have been shown to be effective in reducing oxidative stress, the process of aging, the growth of cancer cells and progression of neurological and neurodegenerative diseases.

3. Return to your previous eating pattern

If you have not obtained any benefits then you may wish to return to your former eating habits. However, if this is the case, do read the section on dietary fats on pages 45 to 49, which presents the latest evidence about the effect of different fats on health status and perhaps take this into consideration when purchasing and consuming meals and snacks.

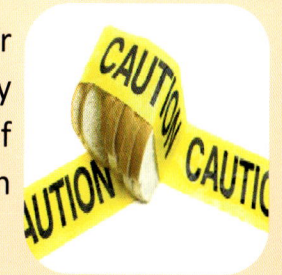

However, if you have experienced benefits then take note that these benefits may disappear once you increase the level of carbohydrate to that consumed previously. Readdress the section on page 9 about the very low carb/high fat lifestyle not being a quick fix. Are you prepared to regain the weight or re-experience symptoms? Being aware of the consequences of your actions will help you make choices regarding your future lifestyle.

www.xperthealth.org.uk

Essential tips to ensure success

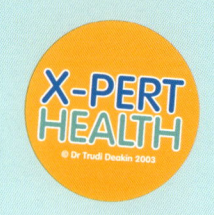

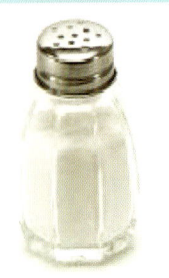

Ensuring adequate mineral intake e.g. salt

Some people in the early weeks after commencing on a very low carb/high fat lifestyle complain of frequent urination, weakness, fatigue, lightheadedness, dizziness, headaches and muscle cramps. These symptoms often result in people giving up but the cause can be easily identified and treated.

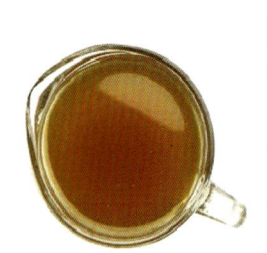

Initially in the first few days an increase in urination occurs when your body is burning up the extra glycogen (stored glucose) in your liver and muscles. Breaking down glycogen releases a lot of water.

Once stored glucose has been used up, circulating insulin levels drop and ketones are produced and this stimulates your kidneys to start excreting excess minerals such as sodium, potassium and magnesium into your urine. This process also results in more frequent urination. Also, you may have dramatically reduced your salt intake by omitting processed foods such as crisps, crackers, bread and cereals.

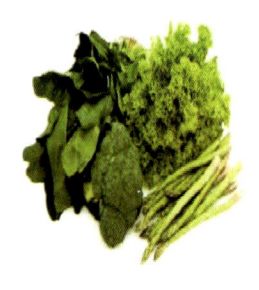

A drop in the blood levels of sodium, potassium and magnesium can lead to you feeling exhausted, lightheaded or dizzy and give you muscle cramps and headaches. This can be avoided and if necessary treated by making sure you obtain sufficient replacement minerals.

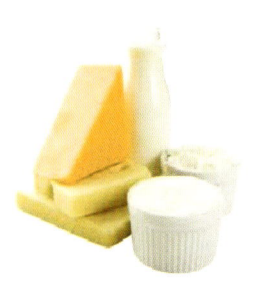

The chemical name for salt is sodium chloride. Although salt has been associated with high blood pressure (hypertension), this occurs in the presence of carb consumption which result in higher circulating levels of insulin. Adding salt to the diet does not lead to hypertension when consuming a very low carb diet especially if your salt intake has dropped by omitting processed foods.

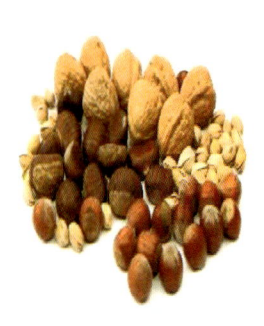

To avoid symptoms of low blood sodium (hyponatremia) it is recommended that you add salt to your meals and/or drink x1 stock cube mixed with hot water each day. Once adapted to the new lifestyle you may find that you no longer need to do this but if you start to experience the symptoms you can easily add more salt to your diet. If you currently have high blood pressure this dietary approach is likely to benefit you but it would be wise to discuss with your healthcare team first (take this handbook with you as they may not be familiar with the very low carb/high fat lifestyle).

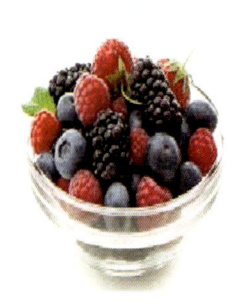

Sufficient amounts of the other minerals such as potassium, magnesium and calcium can be obtained from eating milk and dairy foods, green leafy vegetables, avocado, nuts, berries and dark chocolate that has 70% or higher cocoa content. Some people choose to supplement their diet with mineral supplements but these shouldn't be necessary and it is recommended that you check with your doctor first especially if you have kidney or heart health issues.

www.xperthealth.org.uk

Essential tips to ensure success

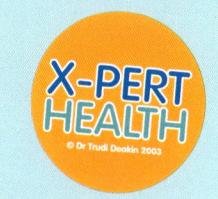

Ensuring sufficient fat intake

If you previously consumed a diet where 50 percent (%) of your calories came from carbohydrate, and you reduce this down to less than 10%, what do you replace those calories with?

We obtain calories from 4 nutrients, fat, protein, carbohydrate and alcohol. Two of these nutrients, fat and protein, are essential to life but we can survive without calories from carbohydrate and alcohol.

Protein should be a central part of a complete diet for adults. While physical growth occurs only for a brief period of life, the need to repair and remodel muscle and bone continues throughout life. For optimal health, maintaining muscle and bone is an critical and essential part of the aging process. Protein needs become more important during periods of reduced food intake such as weight loss or during periods of recovery after illness.

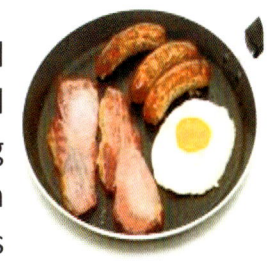

Protein is an important part of good nutrition at every meal. Vitamins and minerals can fulfil nutrient needs on a once-per-day basis but for protein the body has no ability to store a daily supply. To maintain healthy muscles and bones for adults, good sources of protein should be consumed at more than one meal. It is important to eat at least 30g of protein after an overnight fast at breakfast (*break-fast*) to replace the protein used overnight to repair and renew body cells. However, some people prefer not to eat first thing in the morning and breaking the fast can occur at any time throughout the day.

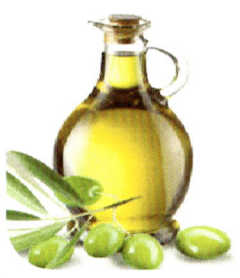

However, although 15-30% of daily calories are required from protein, if it is eaten to excess it is converted to glucose and increases insulin levels. We have already discussed how insulin switches on fat storage and switches off fat burning. Therefore, replacing all carb calories with protein calories is not recommended.

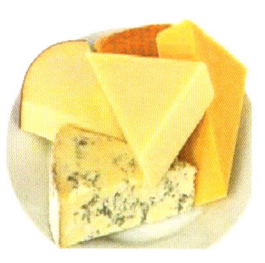

What is effective is replacing carbs with fat. People worry about eating fat, especially saturated fat. See the section on dietary fat (pages 45 to 49) to alleviate any fears. Consuming dietary fat does not cause heart disease and strokes and is necessary to prevent hunger.

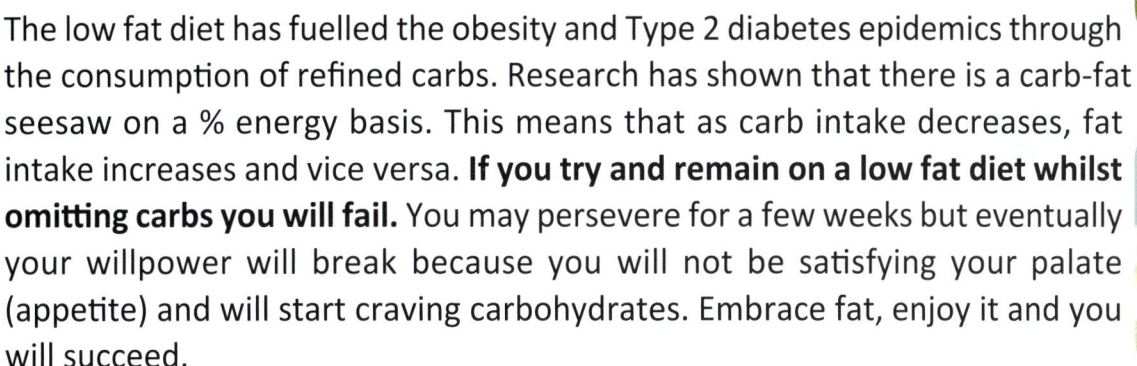

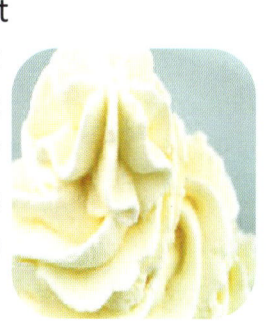

The low fat diet has fuelled the obesity and Type 2 diabetes epidemics through the consumption of refined carbs. Research has shown that there is a carb-fat seesaw on a % energy basis. This means that as carb intake decreases, fat intake increases and vice versa. **If you try and remain on a low fat diet whilst omitting carbs you will fail.** You may persevere for a few weeks but eventually your willpower will break because you will not be satisfying your palate (appetite) and will start craving carbohydrates. Embrace fat, enjoy it and you will succeed.

www.xperthealth.org.uk

Essential tips to ensure success

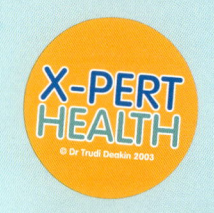

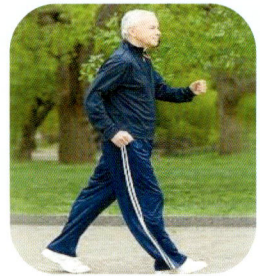

Accepting that physical activity may be more difficult whilst your body is adapting to using fat as its preferred fuel

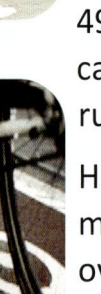

Training the body to rely on fat as fuel instead of carbohydrate is good news for athletes. Even a very lean individual has around 25 times more energy stored as fat than carbohydrate. For example, a 70kg male who has 10% body fat has 49,000 calories of stored energy as fat but only about 2,000 calories stored as carbohydrate. This means that if the body relies on carbohydrate it is going to run out of fuel a lot quicker.

However, becoming keto adapted takes time. What does "Keto-adapted" mean? It is a term used to describe the process whereby a person switches over to using fat almost exclusively for fuel. The brain receives a steady and sustained source of fuel (ketones) thereby protecting the athlete from *hitting the wall* (the term used to describe what happens when the athlete, who is reliant on carbohydrate fuel, runs out of carb stores).

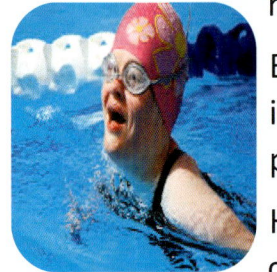

Even if you are not a keen sportsperson, training your body to use fat for energy in preference to carbohydrate will help you to mobilise your fat stores, improve performance and aid recovery. You will become a fat-burning machine!

However, this does not happen immediately when you start on a very low carb/high fat lifestyle, it takes time for your body to adapt. A reduction in your carbohydrate intake to less than 50g per day starts a series of reactions after a few days:

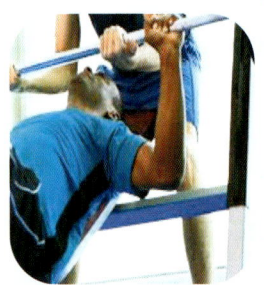

1. The level of insulin in the blood drops significantly
2. You stop converting excess carbs into fat
3. You start breaking down fat stores as an energy source for the body
4. You start converting fat into ketones as an energy source for the brain

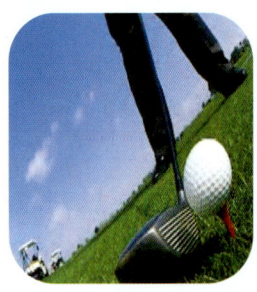

Therefore, during rest or when undertaking low intensity activities, you will probably be obtaining sufficient energy and feel fine. A problem may arise when you try and increase the intensity of exercise. Because it can take up to six weeks for your body to fully adapt from lipogenesis (fat storage) to lipolysis (fat burning), you may struggle to produce adequate energy when the demand increases. This may result in you feeling *heavy legged* with a feeling of exhaustion if you do try to participate in high intensity physical activity.

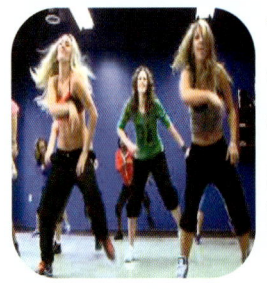

Top tip: Keep with it but don't be too hard on yourself. Slow down, for example, walk or jog instead of running. You will get there eventually (between 2 and 6 weeks) and the day that you can perform once again will be a delight. Most people then find that training becomes easier with better performance and improved recovery times.

www.xperthealth.org.uk

Essential tips to ensure success

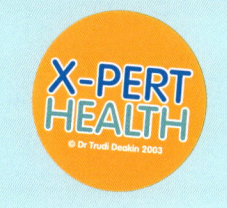

Coping with bad days where you consume too many carbs

We all have bad days so you are not on your own. The trick to success is understanding what went wrong and either accepting it or putting strategies in place to prevent it happening again.

What went wrong?
1. I ate something believing that it didn't contain carbohydrate but then found out it did
2. I gave in to my cravings for some carbohydrate-containing food
3. I attended a family celebration and wanted carbohydrate-rich food such as birthday cake
4. I went out for a meal and there were no low carb options on the menu
5. I had a chaotic day and just had to grab food on the run
6. I went on holiday and didn't want to think about low carb
7. I am an emotional eater and use carbs for comfort depending on my mood (happy, sad, depressed, stressed, upset, excited etc.)

Strategies
1. In the first few months as you become familiar with a very low carb/high fat lifestyle you will eat foods on occasions thinking that they are carb free or low in carbs and then find out they actually do contain carbs. This is a learning curve and you will know next time! Prevention strategies may involve if possible looking on the food packaging nutritional label or checking in carb content books.

2. If you have been craving carb food you need to ask yourself why? The usual reason for this is because you have not been enjoying your new diet. What are the reasons for this? Have you been having enough variety? Have you been eating sufficient fat? You could try to eat a greater variety of foods and also try out some of the recipes (pages 72 to 77) to make substitutes for carbohydrate favourites such as desserts, cakes and biscuits.

3. There will always be temptations especially as life events are often celebrated with cake or other carb-rich foods and drinks. A small piece of cake may contain 30-50g of carbohydrate whereas a larger slice may have 50 to 100g. What are your options? There are five options:
- have a blowout and eat whatever you fancy
- have an ample-sized piece of cake knowing that it will take you above your carb allowance for the day but make sure that everything else you eat is carbohydrate free
- only have a mini portion of cake so that the daily carbs are likely to remain below 50g
- fill up on carb-free foods such as protein with salad and dressings/mayo
- bake a low carb cake (see recipes)

4. If you are eating a meal away from home you may find yourself in a position where there are no low carb options. You can either:
- choose whatever you fancy from the menu knowing that it will take you above your carb-allowance but get back on track afterwards by making sure that you are carb free for the remainder of the day

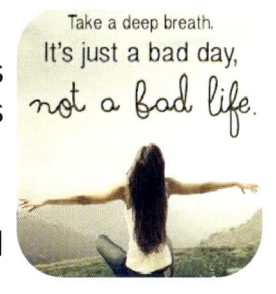

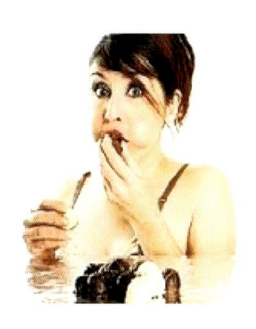

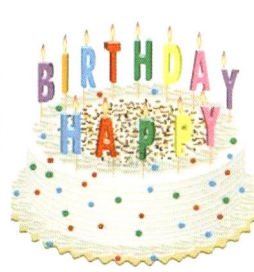

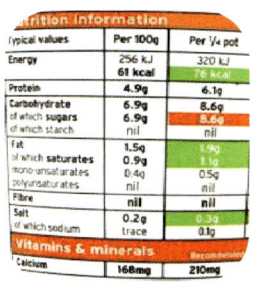

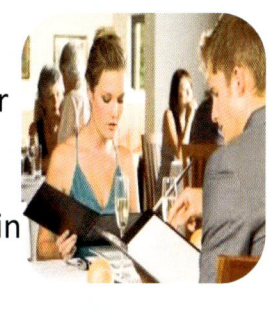

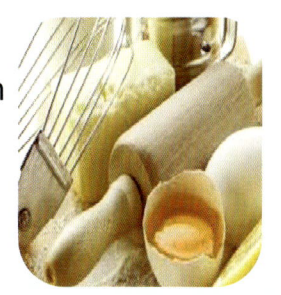

Essential tips to ensure success

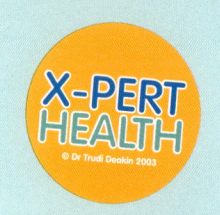

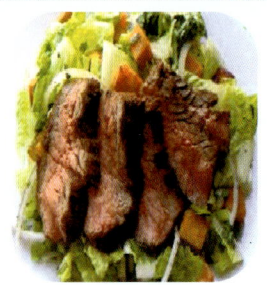

- choose a meal that you know will have fewer carbs or do not eat the carb-rich food on the plate e.g. potato, chips, rice, pasta, bread, chapatti, naan
- ask the waiter if it is possible to replace the carb component with vegetables or salad

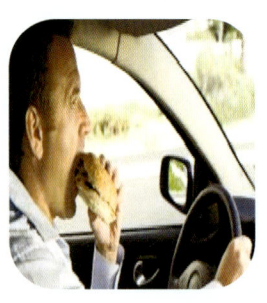

If you are eating at a relative's or a friend's house, you may wish to inform them about your very low carb/high fat lifestyle beforehand. It may become a topic of conversation over dinner as people are often interested to hear more.

5. Many of us have increasingly busy lives but organisation is the key to success. If you know that obtaining the right food will be a challenge, pack a breakfast, lunch or evening meal box and take your food with you (see *suggested meal plans* on pages 69-70 and identify which meals or snacks could be packed in a box to go). Alternately, rather than popping into a bakery to grab a sandwich, pop into a convenience store to purchase cheese or cooked meat, fish or seafood to eat with some cherry tomatoes, cucumber or celery sticks.

6. Going on holiday is something that many of us look forward to. When we do get that much-deserved break, we often wish to relax and leave the day-to-day routine behind. Are you going to leave the lifestyle at home or take it with you? It's not really an approach that you are either "on" or "off" as this can lead to disordered eating and weight gain. Therefore, try to stick to the principles but perhaps be a little more lenient i.e. if you fancy an ice cream, have one but choose small portions and lower carb flavours such as vanilla, chocolate or coconut rather than cookie & cream, rum & raisin or mango. If you do over-consume carbs you may gain weight or become symptomatic but at least you will know why and will be able to get back on track when you return home. Depending on the amount of carbs eaten and the length of the holiday, you may have to go through the adaptation period again.

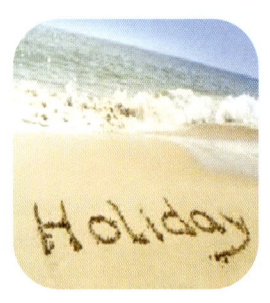

7. Accepting that you are an emotional eater is half the problem solved. The next step is to decide what you are going to do about it. Try keeping a diary to identify your triggers i.e. what emotions lead you to overeat? Now ask yourself, why does this emotion lead me to overeat? The behaviour (eating) is the outcome and you cannot change the eating unless you know what is causing it.

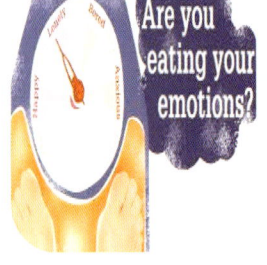

A lot of the time it may be a habit, for example, *"every time I am stressed I reach for the chocolate biscuits"*. It then becomes an association:

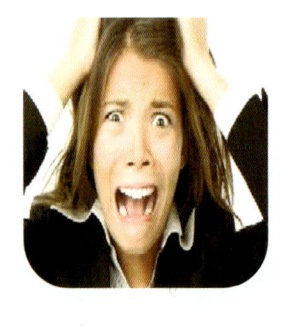

Stress ➡ chocolate biscuits

Breaking that cycle will help you to reduce emotional eating. What could I do when I am stressed that doesn't involve eating? (or at least not eating carb-rich food!). Is it possible for me to replace biscuit eating with a brisk walk in the fresh air? Meeting up with friends? A hot bubble bath in a relaxing environment? A massage? Watching a favourite film?......the options are endless and only you will know what is and isn't possible.

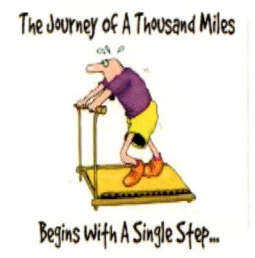

You may identify that you overeat because you feel out of control with your weight or life in general. This feeling of hopelessness may often result in you giving up on your hopes and goals. Try to regain control gradually by setting yourself small and realistic goals. This process will eventually lead to you feeling much more empowered and confident and less likely to use food to try and control your emotions.

www.xperthealth.org.uk

Frequently asked questions

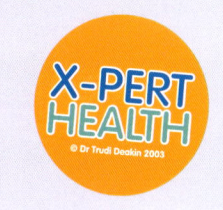

1. I've heard that a low carb diet can lead to constipation, is this true?

Constipation is usually caused by a lack of dietary fibre, insufficient fluid consumption or a sedentary lifestyle. Therefore to prevent constipation, be as active as possible e.g. make sure that you get up and walk around the room every 20 to 30 minutes. Also ensure that you drink enough fluid so that your urine is light coloured. The darker your urine, the more dehydrated you are likely to be. People who follow a very low carb/high fat lifestyle actually tend to eat more fibrous vegetables than they did previously. Although the fibre recommendation in the UK is 18g of fibre per day, the average intake is only 12-15g. You can easily consume 18g of fibre by having 5 to 9 portions of low-carb fruit & vegetables each day. Additional fibre can be obtained by consuming nuts and cooking with ground almonds, coconut and soya flour.

2. I feel shaky and hungry - why is this?

You may have insulin resistance, which means that when you were previously consuming a high carb diet, you were releasing extra insulin from your pancreas into your blood so that you could control blood glucose levels. If you have now dramatically reduced your intake of carbohydrate, it may take a few days for your pancreas to readjust and recognise that you do not require the additional insulin any more.

The high concentration of insulin in your blood may result in your blood glucose levels dropping to a lower level than your body is used to. Don't worry, they will not drop to a level that is dangerous **(unless you are taking certain medication see no. 3 below)** but for a few days until your body has adjusted to your lower blood glucose levels you may experience mild hypoglycaemia "hypo" symptoms such as shakiness, hunger and headaches. Persevere and these symptoms will pass. Do not feel tempted to have a sugary drink or snack as this will once again trigger the release of insulin, which will make the problem worse.

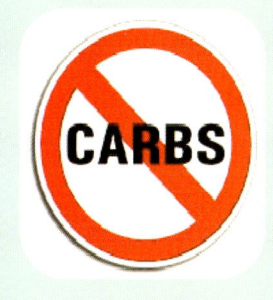

3. Will the low carb high fat lifestyle affect the medication I take?

If you have diabetes and are prescribed a type of medication called sulphonylureas or you are injecting insulin, you will need to discuss a reduction in your medication before you start a very low carb/high fat lifestyle. Examples of sulphonylureas are Gliclazide (Diamicron), Glipizide (Minodiab), Glimepiride (Amaryl), Glibenclamide and Tolbutamide. Sulphonylureas work by stimulating the cells in the pancreas to make more insulin. If you take this medication or inject insulin and reduce your intake of carbohydrate it is likely that blood glucose levels will drop too low and you will experience a much more severe hypo reaction than described in no.2 above.

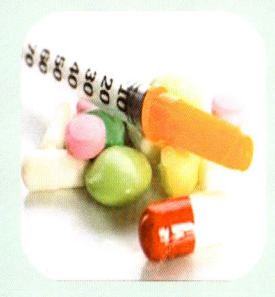

Severe hypos need to be treated with glucose immediately to prevent the brain being starved of glucose and a risk of becoming unconscious. Don't worry, this cannot happen if you do not have diabetes or if your diabetes isn't treated with these medications.

Conditions such as heartburn, blood pressure, blood cholesterol and blood glucose have been shown to improve with a very low carb/high fat lifestyle and you may be able to reduce or even omit medication. Book an appointment with your doctor to review your health results and medication.

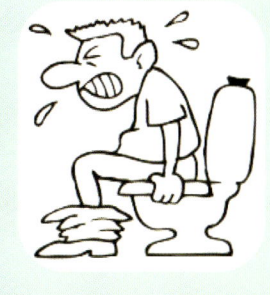

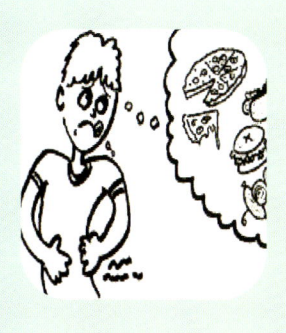

www.xperthealth.org.uk

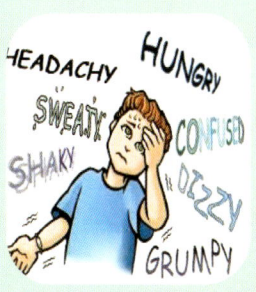

Frequently asked questions

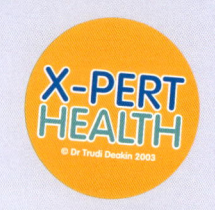

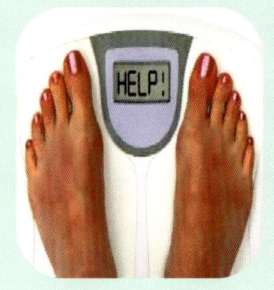

4. I am not losing weight as quickly as I would like. Why is this?

If your purpose for following a very low carb/high fat lifestyle is weight loss but you are losing less than 0.5kg (1lb) per week, or your weight is stable or shock horror, you are gaining weight then you will naturally be very disappointed. Return to Steps 1 to 5. Start by keeping a food diary (Step 1), identify the carbohydrate foods you are eating (Step 2), check that you are eliminating the right foods (Step 3) and you are replacing them with carb-free or very low carb foods (Step 4) and then monitor your intake over a few days (Step 5). Now ask yourself the following questions:

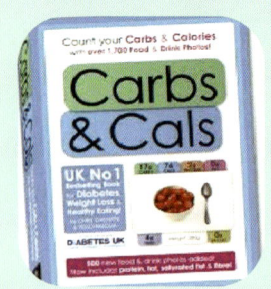

- How many grams of carbs am I eating each day?
- How many calories am I consuming each day?
- How many meals am I having each day?
- How many snacks am I having each day?

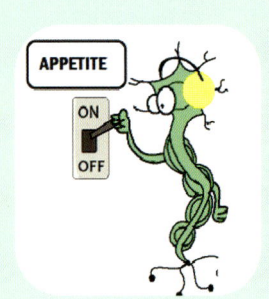

Possible reasons for not achieving weight loss goals

- You are consuming too many carbs. Even if you are consuming less than 50g per day you may be very insulin resistant and therefore need to be stricter and reduce carbs to 20g per day to lose weight.
- A very low carb/high fat lifestyle is more satisfying and although you don't need to count calories, if you override your appetite and eat to excess, you can still gain weight. Ask yourself, am I eating because I am hungry, out of habit *"it's lunchtime therefore I need to eat something"* or *"am I eating to feed my emotions?"*.
- When people learn to read their appetite, they often find that they only need to eat two meals each day. Do you really need snacks? Although nuts are an excellent source of nutrition and can be incorporated into the new lifestyle, many people get into the habit of snacking on them and this is when weight can increase. Weigh a 25g portion of nuts to give you an idea of what 1 portion looks like.

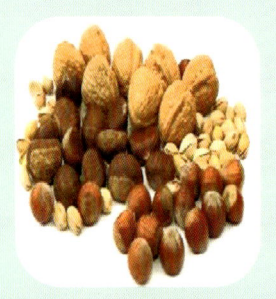

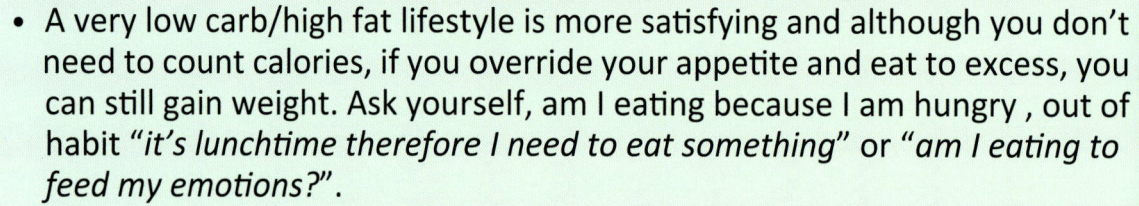

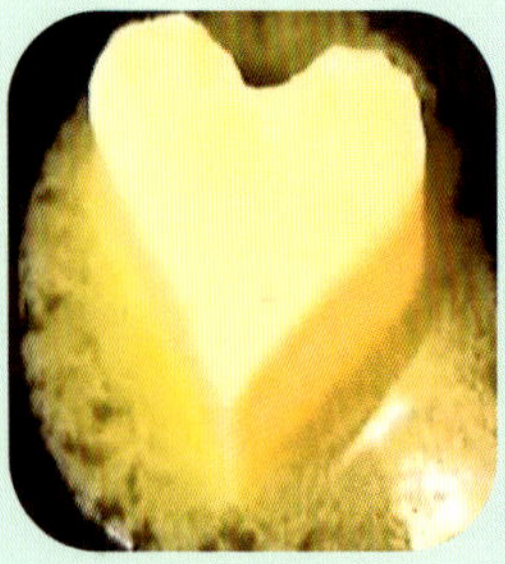

5. I have high cholesterol - will eating more saturated fat increase this?

The biggest myth associated with a very low carb/high fat lifestyle is based on the theory that saturated fat and cholesterol clog up the blood vessels and cause heart disease. There has never been any scientific study which directly proves that cholesterol and saturated fat causes heart disease. Shocking but true.

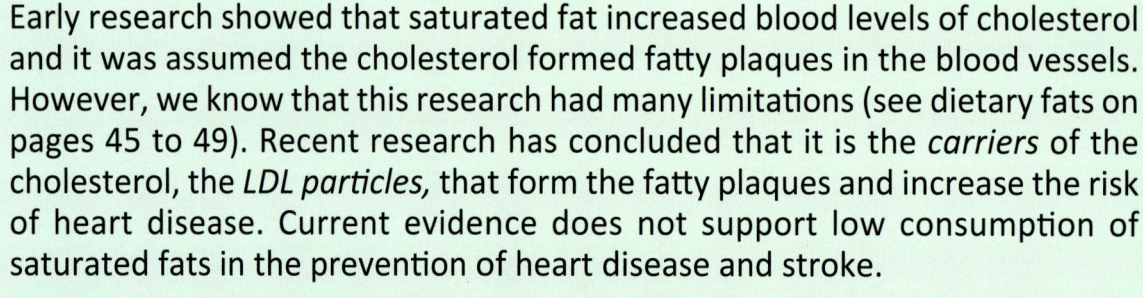

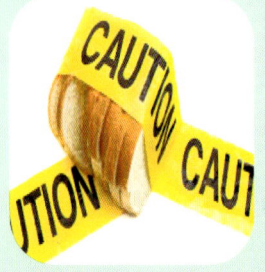

Early research showed that saturated fat increased blood levels of cholesterol and it was assumed the cholesterol formed fatty plaques in the blood vessels. However, we know that this research had many limitations (see dietary fats on pages 45 to 49). Recent research has concluded that it is the *carriers* of the cholesterol, the *LDL particles,* that form the fatty plaques and increase the risk of heart disease. Current evidence does not support low consumption of saturated fats in the prevention of heart disease and stroke.

In contrast, there are several studies showing that a high carbohydrate diet and elevated blood glucose and insulin are highly associated with inflammatory heart disease.

www.xperthealth.org.uk

Frequently asked questions

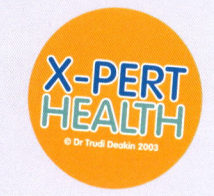

6. Is it OK to follow a low carb high fat dietary approach if I have a medical condition such as diabetes, heart disease, kidney disease or cancer?

If you have a medical condition it is wise to check with your healthcare team before adopting the very low carb/high fat lifestyle. Reducing carbs has been shown to be much more effective than the low fat diet for lowering blood glucose and weight in some people with both Type 1 and Type 2 diabetes but some medications will need to be reduced beforehand (see question 3).

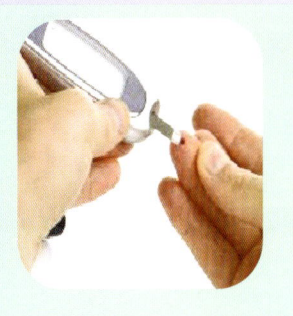

The concern with heart disease is due to the level of dietary fat, especially saturated fat. This issue is discussed in question 5 and it should not be a deterrent for following the very low carb/high fat lifestyle.

The diet is not high protein, it is high fat with moderate protein consumption. If you are healthy with no kidney disease, eating extra protein will not harm your kidneys. However, if you have evidence of kidney disease the traditional advice is to restrict your protein intake. If relevant, restricting protein shouldn't be difficult to do and you can monitor your intake using the tools in Step 5 (pages 20-30).

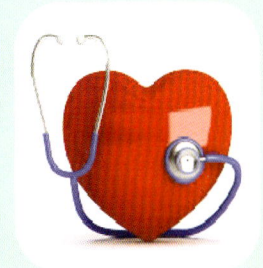

7. I've heard that ketones are dangerous but this diet says that they are good, why?

Healthcare professionals may discourage you from starting on this approach because they believe that ketones are bad for you. This is totally understandable because they have seen people with Type 1 diabetes suffer from a condition called ketoacidosis. This usually only occurs in people with Type 1 diabetes who have a severe deficiency in insulin. The result is extremely high blood glucose levels, ketone levels that are 10-fold above the levels produced from dietary ketosis and severe dehydration from the kidneys trying to flush the glucose and ketones out in the urine. *Diabetic ketoacidosis and dietary ketosis are completely different conditions.*

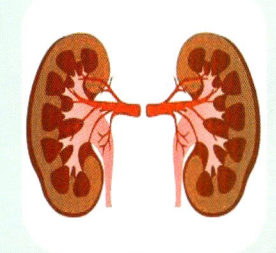

Normal dietary ketosis is NOT dangerous. Every person goes into mild ketosis each time they go without eating for 6-8 hours. Children and pregnant women frequently produce ketones as they use up their energy stores more quickly. Have you ever smelt the breath of children first thing in the morning? It often smells like pear drops. This is the ketones. Clearly dietary ketosis is not harmful as long as some insulin is circulating within the body and blood glucose levels remain in the normal range. In fact, emerging research is providing evidence that dietary ketosis may be benefical as a treatment for inflammation, aging, neurological and neurodegenerative diseases and cancer.

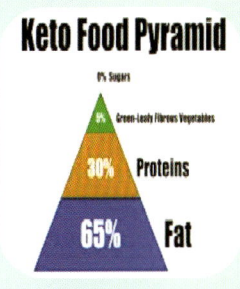

8. What about raspberry ketone supplements, will they help me to lose weight?

Raspberry ketone is the compound that gives raspberries their strong aroma and flavour. A synthetic version of it is used in cosmetics, processed foods and weight loss supplements. Some studies in mice and rats show that raspberry ketones can protect against weight gain and fatty liver. However, these studies used massive dosages, much higher than you would get with a supplement. There is currently no evidence that raspberry ketone supplements can cause weight loss in humans. It is therefore better to produce ketones naturally in your body by adopting a very low carb/high fat lifestyle.

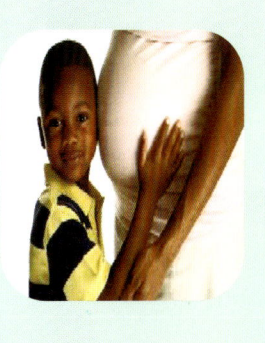

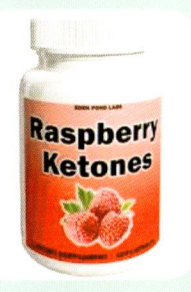

www.xperthealth.org.uk

Frequently asked questions

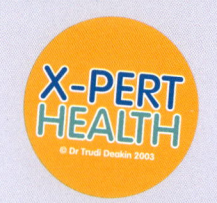

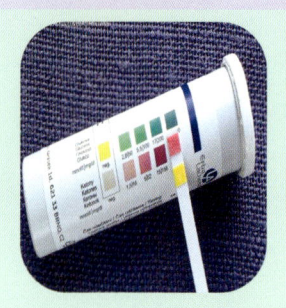

9. How do I know what level of ketone I am producing? Can I measure them?

If you are achieving your goal(s) with your new lifestyle it is unlikely that testing ketone levels will bring an additional benefit. However if you would like to monitor levels of ketones there are three ways to test:
- urine test strips
- home blood meters
- breath test meters

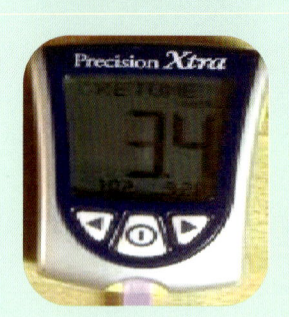

Ketones can be tested using urine test strips which measure the level of a ketone called acetoacetate in the urine. However, once your body has adapted to burning fat for energy urine testing is not as accurate as you will have a greater blood concentration of another ketone called beta-hydroxybutyrate (BHB). Many home blood meters will measure levels of BHB and although the meters are inexpensive, the test strips are pricey. The breath test measures ketones in the breath (acetone). More information is available on our website.

10. Does the very low carb/high fat lifestyle cause bad breath?

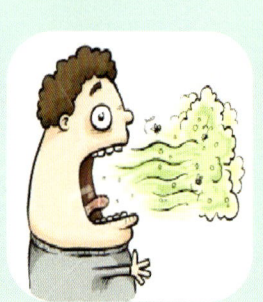

One of the results of cutting carbs is that we start to use more fat for energy generating ketones. One type of ketone, acetone, tends to be excreted in urine and in the breath. The description of the smell varies but it is often described as "fruity" or like the smell of peardrops. The good news is that keto-breath usually doesn't last forever. Most people find it dies down after a few weeks as they adapt to using the ketones for energy (see above). There are things you can do to minimise the impact of "keto-breath":
- Drink more water
- Use natural breath fresheners such as mint, parsley, cloves, cinnamon and fennel seeds
- Try breath capsules which are usually made from parsley oil e.g. Mint Asure. Some people swear by them whereas others find they do not help.
- Try sugar-free mints or gum

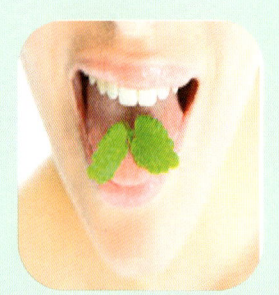

11. I feel really tired, is this normal?

Whilst your body is adapting to using fat as its preferred fuel rather than carbohydrate you may feel a little more tired than you usually do. This is because your body will have used up its glucose stores and will not be used to solely relying on fat and ketones for energy. However this will be short-lived and after a week or two you will probably find that your energy levels improve considerably. Many people report feeling much more energetic than they did before. This is because fat can provide vast amounts of energy compared to carbohydrate. Even a lean person could have energy stores that are 25-fold whereas these could be 500-fold for an obese individual.

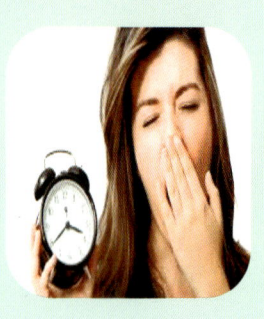

12. Is the diet nutritionally complete or do I need to take supplements?

Critics of the very low carb/high fat lifestyle often state that it will result in being deficient in vitamin C and the B vitamins but as long as you are eating a good variety of food i.e. natural fats (butter, lard, olive oil, coconut oil), meats, poultry, fish, leafy green vegetables, nuts and berries, you will probably be consuming more vitamins and minerals than you did on your previous diet and there will be no need for supplements. This is a good thing as some studies have shown that taking vitamin tablets can be harmful to health.

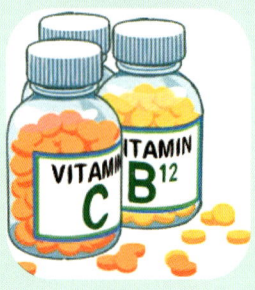

www.xperthealth.org.uk

Frequently asked questions

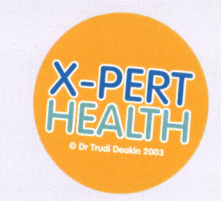

13. Is it possible to be gluten/wheat/lactose free?

Absolutely. This is good news for people with coeliac disease (a lifelong auto-immune disease caused by intolerance to gluten), dermatitis herpetiformis (a skin condition linked to coeliac disease) and intolerances to wheat and lactose that are becoming much more prevalent.

Gluten is a protein found in wheat, rye and barley and a similar protein is found in oats. All of these grains belong in the carbohydrate section of the Nutrition for Health plate. The very low carb/high fat lifestyle is gluten and wheat-free as these carbohydrate-rich grains tend to be omitted when carbs are restricted to less than 50g per day. Flour substitutes, such as ground almonds, coconut and soya flour, that do not contain gluten can be used to make bread, scones, pastry, cakes and biscuits.

Lactose intolerance is a common digestive problem where the body is unable to digest lactose, a type of sugar mainly found in milk and dairy products. A major source of lactose is milk (cow, goat and sheep) and products made from milk such as butter, cream, ice cream, cream cheese and milk chocolate. Some dairy products however, such as hard cheese and yogurt, contain lower levels of lactose than milk.

Depending on how severe your lactose intolerance is you may need to change the amount of milk in your diet. This should be easier as:

- breakfast cereals are omitted
- cream contains less lactose and can replace milk in drinks and sauces
- calcium requirements can be achieved from eating full fat yogurt and hard cheese
- processed food with hidden sources of milk/milk products are reduced
- you can also purchase unsweetened milk made from soya, almonds, hazelnuts and coconut.

14. Is this not just another fad diet?

The majority of diets are marketed purely as a weight loss solution and work solely because they lead to a reduced intake of calories. The low fat diet is an example of this. The amount of calories per gram of fat is greater than any other of the nutrients (fat = 9kcal; alcohol = 7kcal; protein = 4kcal; carbs = 4kcal) and therefore it makes sense that if you cut the fat, you will also cut the calories. However, major flaws are present with this hypothesis:

- Fat increases the satiety value of a meal i.e. without fat the appetite is less likely to be satisfied
- As the calories from fat reduce, calories from carbohydrate increase. Carbs stimulate the weight-promoting hormone, insulin, that switches on fat storage and switches off fat burning in the body.

Therefore low fat diets are often doomed to fail and then it is only a matter of time before the diet is broken and people return to their old style of eating. These diets have fuelled the obesity and Type 2 diabetes epidemics. The low carb high fat lifestyle is not a fad, it is a style of eating that can be adopted for life to not only support people obtaining and maintaining a healthy body weight but also prevent and treat a whole host of other conditions.

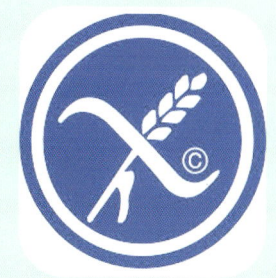

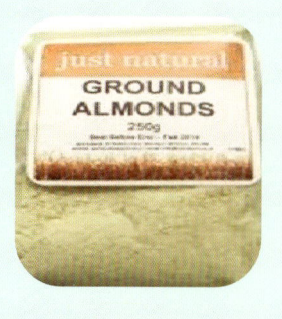

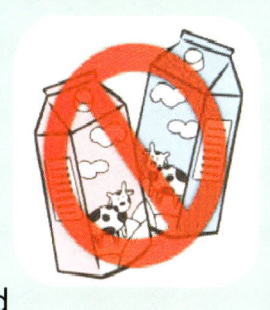

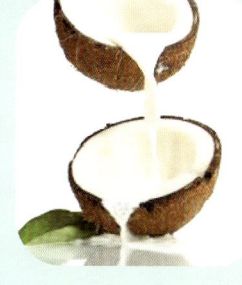

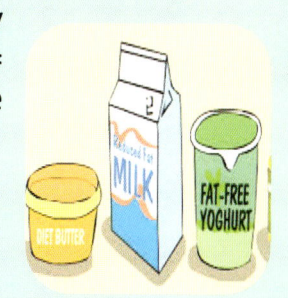

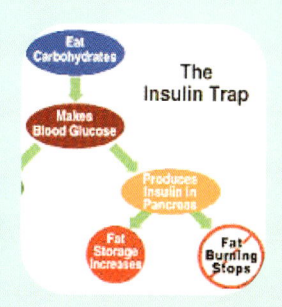

www.xperthealth.org.uk

Frequently asked questions

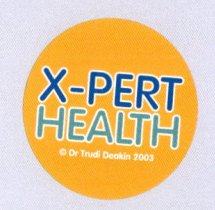

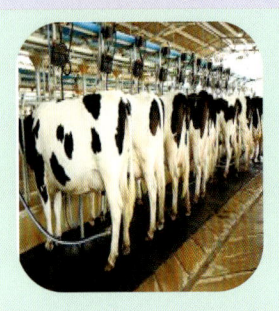

15. What about red meat? Isn't it bad for me?

Red meat is one of the most controversial foods in the history of nutrition. Despite the fact that humans have been eating it throughout evolution, many people believe that it can cause harm. Traditional populations like the Inuit and Masai have eaten lots of meat, much more than the average Westerner, but remained in excellent health.

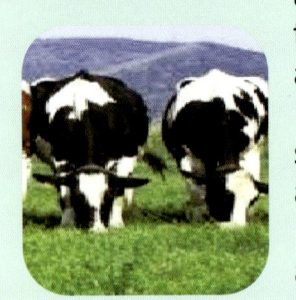

However, the meat we eat today is vastly different from the meat our ancestors ate when animals roamed free and ate grass. It is important when examining the health effects of meat to realise it depends how the animals have been fed and treated.

- **Processed meat.** These products go through various processing methods such as smoking and curing. They are then treated with nitrates, preservatives and various chemicals. Examples include sausages and bacon
- **Red meat.** Conventional red meats are fairly unprocessed, but the cattle are usually factory farmed. Meats that are red when raw are defined as "red" meats. Examples are lamb, beef, pork and offal
- **White meat.** Meats that are white when cooked are defined as "white" meats. Examples include chicken and turkey
- **Grass-fed organic meat.** This meat comes from animals that have been naturally fed, raised organically and not been given drugs and hormones. They also don't have any artificial chemicals added to them

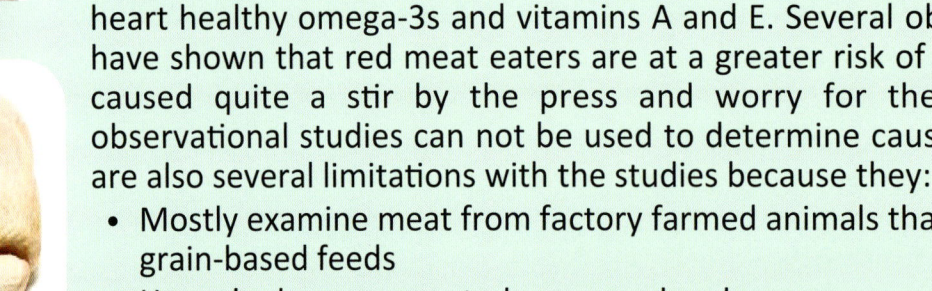

Red meat is very nutritious. It's a great source of protein, iron, B12, zinc, creatine and various other nutrients. Grass-fed meat also contains plenty of heart healthy omega-3s and vitamins A and E. Several observational studies have shown that red meat eaters are at a greater risk of cancer and this has caused quite a stir by the press and worry for the public. However, observational studies can not be used to determine cause and effect. There are also several limitations with the studies because they:

- Mostly examine meat from factory farmed animals that have been fed grain-based feeds
- Haven't always separated processed and non-processed meat
- Rely on food frequency questionnaires which are not the most accurate way to assess an individuals food intake
- Contain many confounding factors. For example, because the red meat message has been around for years, it has been shown that people who have eaten more red meat over the last couple of decades tend to be less health conscious and more likely to smoke, drink excessively, eat more sugar and be less active

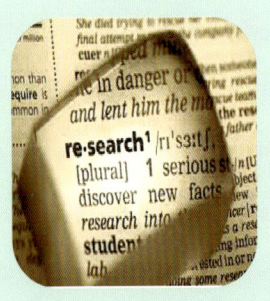

Clinical trials are much higher quality studies and although none have been done directly looking at intakes of red meat, trials on low-fat diets (low in red meat) don't show a reduction in cancer and trials on low-carb diets (high in red meat) almost invariably lead to improved health outcomes.

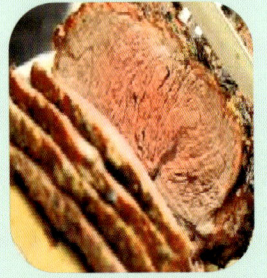

When you look past the scare tactics and sensationalist headlines, you realise that there are no controlled trials linking red meat to disease in humans. As long as you're choosing unprocessed (preferably grass-fed) red meat and make sure to use gentler cooking methods to avoid burnt or charred pieces, then there is probably nothing to worry about.

www.xperthealth.org.uk

Frequently asked questions

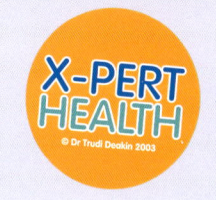

16. I have heard that coffee can increase blood glucose levels, should I stop drinking it?

Coffee is the most recognisable, widely consumed and readily available non-alcoholic beverage in the world, coming in many varieties and ways of preparations. Caffeine, which is a naturally-occurring substance with a bitter taste, stimulates the central nervous system, making you feel more alert. In moderate doses, it can actually offer health benefits, including boosts to memory, concentration and mental health. Any protective effects of coffee are unlikely to be solely effects of caffeine, but rather, a broader range of chemical constituents present such as magnesium, lignans and chlorogenic acids.

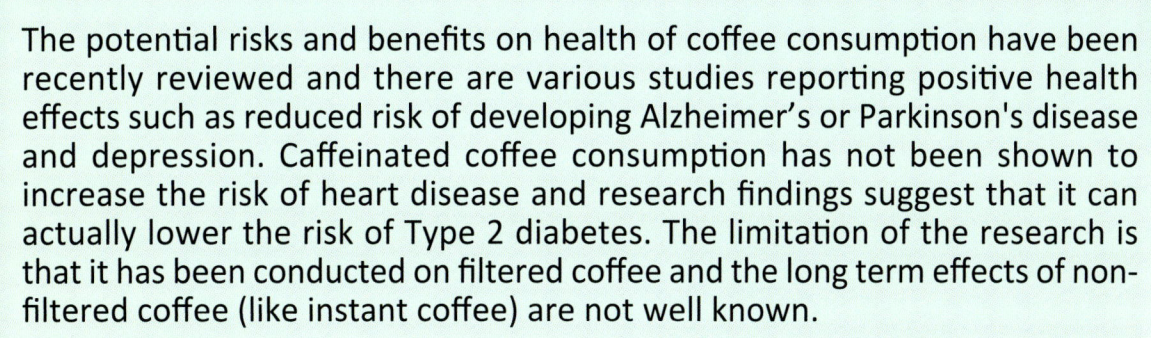

The potential risks and benefits on health of coffee consumption have been recently reviewed and there are various studies reporting positive health effects such as reduced risk of developing Alzheimer's or Parkinson's disease and depression. Caffeinated coffee consumption has not been shown to increase the risk of heart disease and research findings suggest that it can actually lower the risk of Type 2 diabetes. The limitation of the research is that it has been conducted on filtered coffee and the long term effects of non-filtered coffee (like instant coffee) are not well known.

The reason why some earlier observational studies reported an association between coffee consumption and increased risk of heart disease may be related to some unfavourable lifestyle behaviours that are often associated with coffee, e.g. smoking. However, for some individuals, excess amounts of caffeine can trigger a fast heart rate, insomnia, anxiety and restlessness among other side effects and for these people, abstinence or opting for decaffeinated may be preferable.

Although more research on the health effect of coffee is needed to formulate sound recommendations on its consumption, current information suggests that coffee is not as bad as we were told and there is no need to stop drinking it if you do not experience any ill effects.

However, take note:
- abruptly stopping caffeine-containing coffee drinking can sometimes lead to symptoms of withdrawal, including headaches and irritability
- a latte or cappuccino can contain around 20g carbohydrate due to the milk

17. I have heard that coconut oil is good for you, is this correct?

Yes. Plenty of populations around the world have thrived for generations eating massive amounts of coconut. Its unique combination of fatty acids can have profoundly positive effects on health. The benefits include:
- medium chain triglycerides (MCTs) that are rapidly turned into ketones and increase the amount of fat you burn
- substances that help to kill harmful bacteria preventing infections
- a significantly reduced appetite
- improvement in blood fat levels
- the option to use it as an effective skin moisturizer, mouthwash, hair conditioner and mild sunscreen
- providing a possible treatment for neurological and neurodegenerative diseases by supplying brain cells with ketones

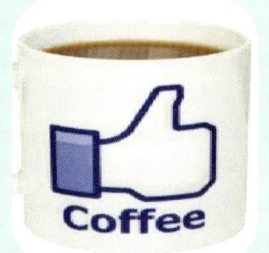

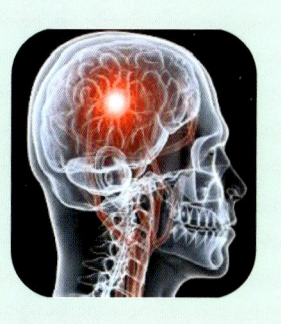

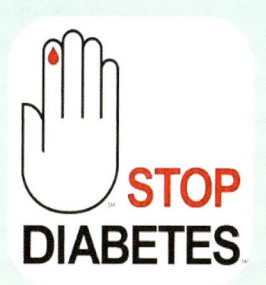

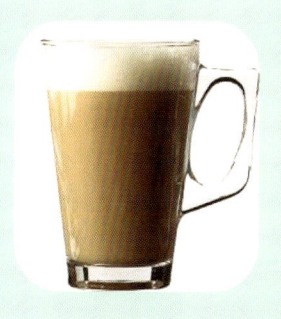

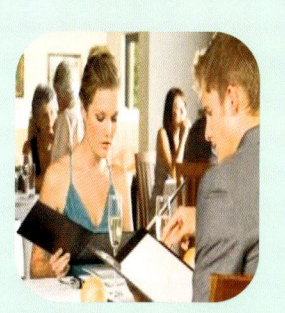

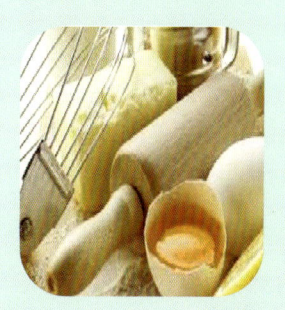

www.xperthealth.org.uk

Frequently asked questions

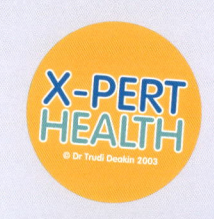

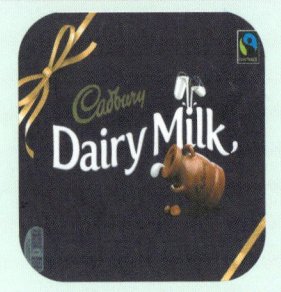

18. I am really missing chocolate. Are there any types that I can eat?

Dark chocolate is loaded with nutrients. It is one of the best sources of antioxidants and minerals such as iron, magnesium, potassium, zinc and selenium. It is also a great source of fibre. However, it is high in calories and it does contain carbs so it is best consumed in moderation. The table below compares different varieties of chocolate. Always check the label as different brands can contain very different concentrations of carbohydrate.

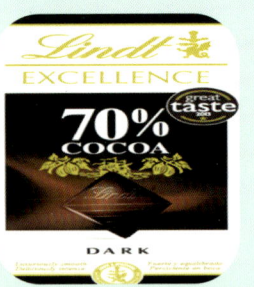

Per 100g	White chocolate (Green & Blacks)	Milk chocolate (Dairy Milk)	70% cocoa chocolate (Lindt)	70% cocoa chocolate (Green & Blacks)	85% cocoa chocolate (Lindt)	85% cocoa chocolate (Green & Blacks)	90% cocoa chocolate (Lindt)	99% cocoa chocolate (Lindt)	Diabetic chocolate (Boots)
Calories (kcal)	580	530	566	580	584	630	580	590	482
Carbs (g)	51	57	34	37	19	23	14	8	17*
Sugar (g)	51	56	29	29	14	14	7	1	11
Fat (g)	39	31	41	42	46	54	55	51	34
Saturated fat (g)	23	19	24	25	28	32	30	30	21
Fibre (g)	0	1	12	10	16	12	13	20	3

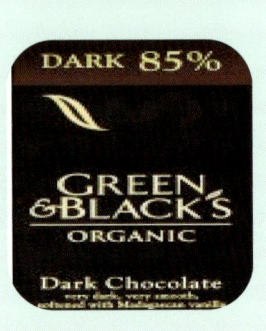

*The nutritional label for the diabetic chocolate states 49.7g carbohydrates per 100g but 33g are polyols which are unavailable carbs and therefore the amount of available carbohydrate is 17g per 100 bar.

The fats in cocoa and dark chocolate are mostly saturated and monounsaturated, which supports the high fat lifestyle. Flavanols help to dilate the blood vessels, which improves blood flow reducing blood pressure.

Clinical studies have shown that dark chocolate with a high percentage of cocoa solids can improve several important risk factors to prevent heart disease:
- the antioxidants in the chocolate prevent LDLs (the particles in the blood that carry cholesterol) from oxidising. This then prevents fatty plaque formation in the blood vessels
- HDL particles (that carry cholesterol back to the liver so that they can be excreted from the body) are increased
- insulin resistance is reduced

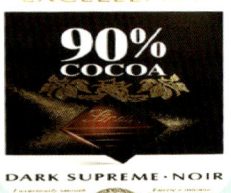

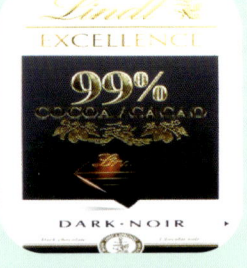

The bioactive compounds in dark chocolate may also be great for your skin and can protect against sun-induced damage, improve blood flow to the skin and increase skin density and hydration. Finally, chocolate may improve brain function as it increases blood flow to the brain.

But of course, as stated above, this doesn't mean people should eat it to excess as it is still high in calories. Maybe have a square or two after dinner and attempt to eat it slowly so that you can savour the intense flavour.

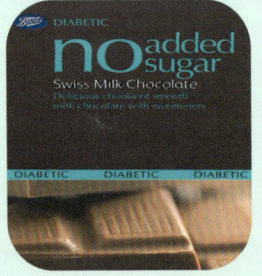

If you do not like dark chocolate, you could try diabetic chocolate. The example on the left displays in the nutritional label that it has 49.7g carbs per 100g, but it only has 17g of available carbs as it contains a type of unavailable carbohydrate called polyols. Always check the label! This will be explained in the section on sweeteners on page 52 to 54.

www.xperthealth.org.uk

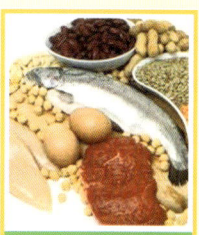

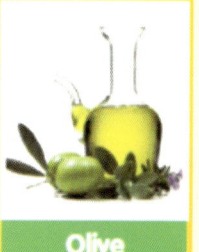

Filling up on fat

Fat is essential to life. There are several different types of fat and they all have different properties and functions in the body, some beneficial and some detrimental. Foods contain a variety of the different fats but often one type predominates.

Trans fats are found in hydrogenated vegetable oil. Baked goods (especially doughnuts, cookies, cakes, chips and crackers) and deep-fried foods are more likely to contain the hydrogenated fat that gives rise to trans fats. They are harmful because they have been shown to increase risk of heart disease. Those most at risk from trans fats are people eating deep-fried takeaway food regularly and/or purchasing cheaper or foreign brands of processed food. These foods also tend to be higher in carbs, which can be converted to fat in the liver.

Saturated fat is found in meat, eggs, dairy foods, butter, lard, cheese, cream and coconut oil. Foods that contain large amounts of saturated fat are more likely to be hard at room temperature. Previously thought to increase cholesterol levels and contribute to heart disease, this diet-heart hypothesis has never been proven. Recent research has concluded that current evidence does not support low consumption of saturated fats in the prevention of heart disease and stroke.

Dietary cholesterol is found in animal products such as eggs, liver, kidneys and shellfish. Cholesterol is essential in the body. It is a waxy, fat-like substance that performs five main functions: it helps make the outer coating of body cells; it makes up the bile acids that work to digest food in the gut; it allows the body to make Vitamin D; hormone production, like oestrogen in women and testosterone in men; it is essential for brain function. Without cholesterol, none of these functions would take place, and without these functions, human beings wouldn't exist.

Polyunsaturated fat. There are 2 types: **Omega-6 fats** are found in seeds and oils like sunflower, safflower, sesame, corn & soya. **Omega-3 fats** are found in oily fish such as salmon, mackerel and sardines, nuts, cold-pressed rapeseed oil, flaxseeds and chia seeds, some pulses, tofu, free-range eggs and grass-fed cattle. A small amount of both are essential for health because they cannot be made by the human body. However, the ratio between omega-6 and omega-3 fats is currently too high due to the excessive intake of refined vegetable oils. Too many omega-6s increase oxidation and inflammation. Readdressing the balance, by omitting refined vegetable oils and ensuring sufficient intake of omega-3, is beneficial for health.

Monounsaturated fat. A good source is olive oil*. It is also found in peanut or groundnut oil; nuts such as peanuts, almonds, cashews, brazil nuts; meat; avocados. Monounsaturated fat protects against cell damage because it is less prone to oxidation and free radical damage.

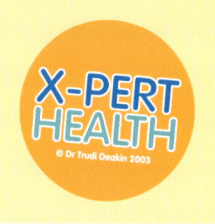

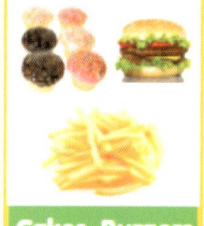

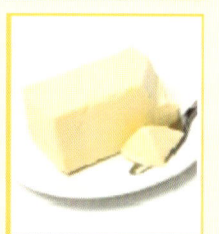

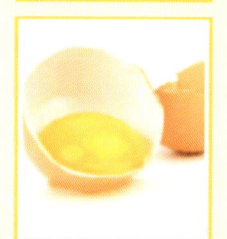

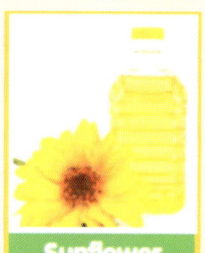

*Extra Virgin is best because heat and chemicals have not been used to extract the oil.

www.xperthealth.org.uk

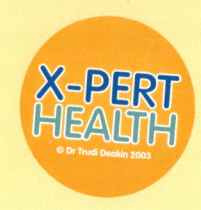

Filling up on fat

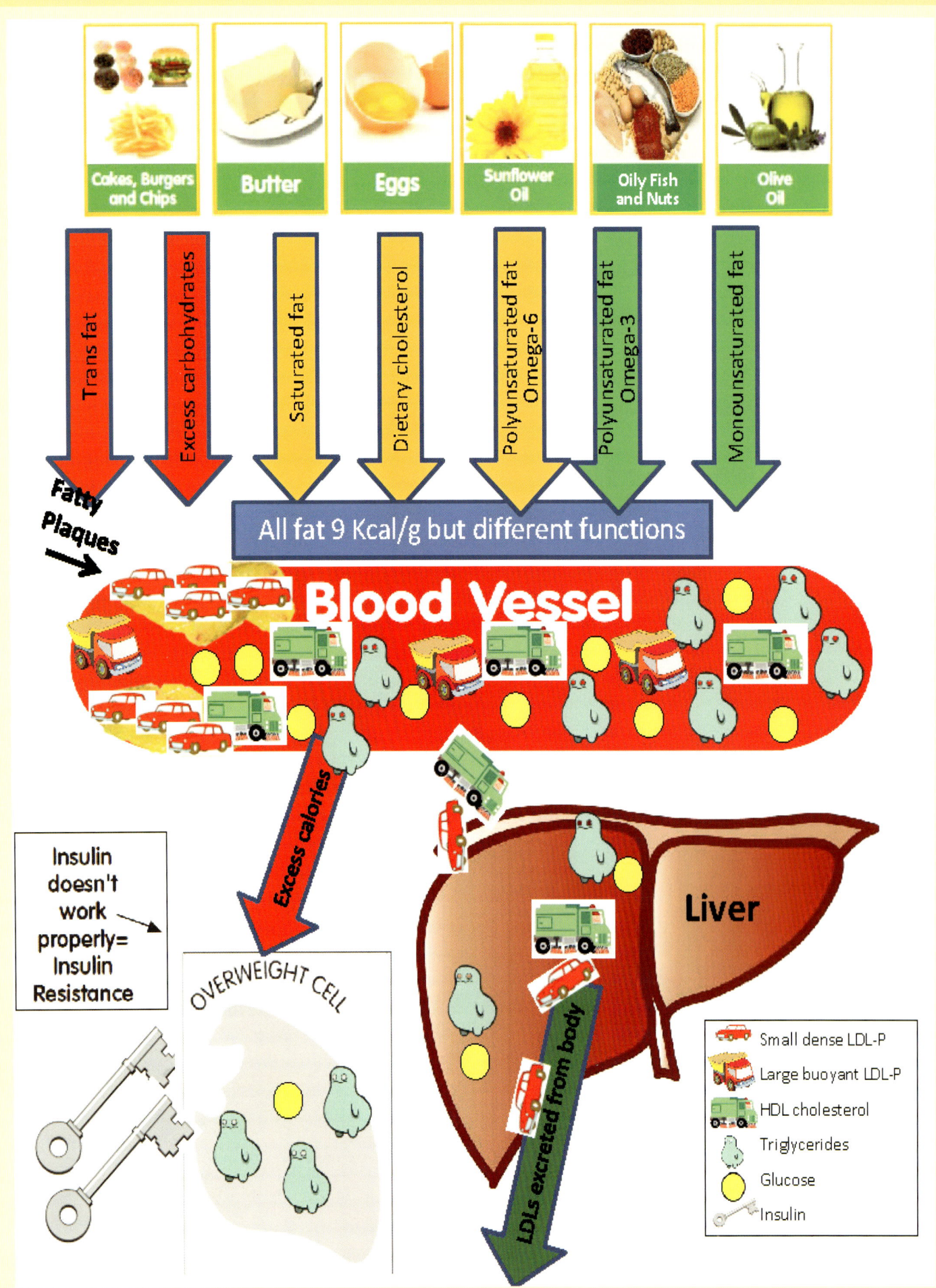

Cakes, Burgers and Chips	Butter	Eggs	Sunflower Oil	Oily Fish and Nuts	Olive Oil
Trans fat / Excess carbohydrates	Saturated fat	Dietary cholesterol	Polyunsaturated fat Omega-6	Polyunsaturated fat Omega-3	Monounsaturated fat

All fat 9 Kcal/g but different functions

Fatty Plaques →

Blood Vessel

Excess calories → OVERWEIGHT CELL

Insulin doesn't work properly = Insulin Resistance

Liver

LDLs excreted from body

Legend:
- Small dense LDL-P
- Large buoyant LDL-P
- HDL cholesterol
- Triglycerides
- Glucose
- Insulin

www.xperthealth.org.uk

Filling up on fat

Dispelling the myth that saturated fat is bad for you

Contrary to the traditional viewpoint, we now know that saturated fat does not increase risk of cardiovascular disease (heart disease and stroke). This incorrect theory was generated following the 1958 Seven Countries Study, which examined the association between diet and cardiovascular disease in different countries and concluded that fat, especially saturated fat caused heart disease. The results have been widely cited and have crucially influenced dietary guidelines and industrial practices all over the world.

However, this study was an observational study with severe methodological limitations, such as: collecting data during periods of Lent when people were abstaining from meat, fish, dairy products, eggs and cheese; not choosing countries where people eat a lot of fat but have little heart disease (such as France and Switzerland) and countries where fat consumption is low but the rate of heart disease is high (such as Chile); not assessing sugar and refined carbohydrate intakes although these had increased substantially post war; only analysing the nutritional intake of 4% of the study participants.

Although low fat and low saturated fat diets have been the cornerstone of dietary recommendations since 1983, saturated fat has never been proven to be the culprit of heart disease in clinical trials. It has recently been acknowledged that current evidence does not support guidelines that encourage high consumption of polyunsaturated fat and low consumption of saturated fat for the prevention and treatment of cardiovascular disease.

Facts about cardiovascular disease

1. Cardiovascular disease (CVD) is a general term that describes a disease of the heart or blood vessels. A build-up of fatty plaques and prolonged inflammation damages the walls of the blood vessels causing them to harden and narrow (atherosclerosis) or blood clots to form (thrombosis). This results in reduced blood flow around the body especially to the heart and brain.

2. Cholesterol has been blamed for causing CVD. As stated on page 45, cholesterol is essential to life, we would die without it. Your body can make all the cholesterol it needs. It is also found in some foods but it is poorly absorbed from the digestive system. If cholesterol is absorbed, your body just makes less of it.

3. Cholesterol needs to be transported to every cell in the body via the blood. As a fat, cholesterol cannot dissolve in blood and therefore needs to be carried. The transport vehicles designed for this purpose are special fatty proteins called LDLs. These carriers are frequently referred to as cholesterol but this is incorrect, they are proteins that carry the cholesterol in the blood. LDLs come in different sizes and ideally these transporters should be large (like trucks). People who eat excess carbohydrate tend to have an abundance of small LDL transporters (like cars) to carry the required amount of cholesterol.

4. Let's relate blood vessels to roads. Trucks carry goods, and in this case, the goods are cholesterol. The more traffic there is on the roads, the more accidents there will be. It is no different within the body's blood vessels. The more numerous small LDLs (cars) instead of large LDLs (trucks) leads to more crashes where LDLs embed themselves into the blood vessel wall, causing inflammation and dropping the goods (cholesterol) they were carrying. The cholesterol is merely the innocent back-seat passenger! Large LDLs (trucks) are much more stable and are therefore less likely to cause the fatty plaques and inflammation that leads to heart disease.

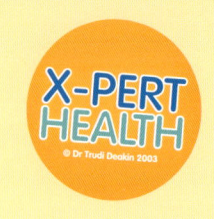

Filling up on fat

5. HDL is another cholesterol transporter which is frequently termed 'good' or 'healthy' because instead of transporting cholesterol to the cells, it acts as a road sweeper mopping up as much excess cholesterol as it can. The excess cholesterol is then taken back to the liver where it is excreted or recycled. Another benefit of HDL is that it contains antioxidant molecules that can prevent small LDL particles from being oxidised i.e. the road sweepers spray a protective coating on the LDL transporters to stop them from rusting. These actions are thought to explain why high levels of HDL are associated with low risk of heart disease. Eating carbohydrate to excess can result in low levels of the beneficial HDL particles.

6. If there are too many small LDLs or not enough HDLs, the fatty plaques can increase in size, harden or rupture (break open). Hardened plaque narrows the coronary arteries (blood vessels around the heart) and reduces the flow of oxygen-rich blood to the heart. This can cause chest pain or discomfort called angina.

7. If the plaque ruptures, blood cell fragments may clump together to form blood clots. Blood clots can further narrow the coronary arteries and worsen angina. If a clot becomes large enough, it can mostly or completely block a coronary artery and cause a heart attack.

Summary: There is insufficient evidence for concluding that dietary saturated fat is associated with an increased risk of CVD. Many recent studies have looked into the importance of LDL-particle size and have concluded that people whose LDL particles are predominantly small and dense have a threefold greater risk of coronary heart disease. This could explain why some individuals with high cholesterol don't experience heart problems but why some with low cholesterol levels do.

How the diet can influence risk of CVD

The diagram on page 46 demonstrates how your diet can influence your CVD risk.

Red light - avoid

Trans fats increase levels of small dense LDL particles. Both observational studies and clinical trials have found that trans fats significantly increase your risk of heart disease. Consumption of trans fats has gone down significantly in recent years. However, current intake is still high enough to cause harm. In order to avoid trans fats, the best thing you can do is eliminate processed foods from your diet.

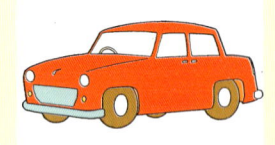

Eating carbohydrates to excess increases levels of both blood triglyceride levels and small dense LDL particles. This process is called de novo lipogenesis, which basically means that the excess calories from carbohydrate are converted to fat.

Amber light - in moderation

Saturated fat and dietary cholesterol are not detrimental to health unless eaten to excess leading to weight gain. However, despite the higher calorie content, eating high-fat products is NOT associated with obesity but is associated with many health benefits. One of these is that saturated fat has been shown to increase levels of the HDL particles that have been shown to be protective against CVD.

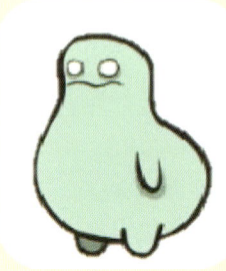

Small dense LDL

Triglycerides

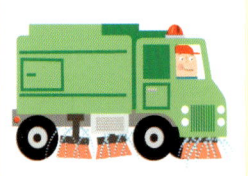

Protective HDL

Filling up on fat

A small amount of **omega-6 polyunsaturated fat** is essential for life but there are two reasons why it should only be eaten in moderation.

It is very unstable and prone to oxidisation resulting in the formation of free radicals, which is bad news in the body as they attack body cells increasing risk of heart disease and cancer.

Omega-6s are also pro-inflammatory which means that they encourage chronic inflammation in the body, which is the starting point for many diseases. Therefore the use of vegetable oils is discouraged.

What are Free radicals?

Free radicals are like robbers which are deficient in energy.

Free radicals attack and snatch energy from the other cells to satisfy themselves.

Green light - eat freely

Omega-3 polyunsaturated fats are anti-inflammatory. The omega-6 and omega-3 ratio is currently 16:1. Reducing this ratio to a recommended 4:1 has been associated with improvements in health outcomes in conditions such as CVD, arthritis and cancer.

Monounsaturated fat is the predominant fat in both olive oil and rapeseed oil. Research looking at the benefits of olive oil has shown it to lower blood pressure, protect LDL particles from oxidation, reduce inflammation and help prevent unwanted blood clotting. N.B. olive and rapeseed oils need to be cold pressed i.e. extra virgin, as refining using heat and solvents create the detrimental trans fats discussed on page 48. In the UK, vegetable oil is usually refined rapeseed oil.

How does the low fat diet increase risk of obesity, Type 2 diabetes, CVD and fatty liver?

1. *Cell damage.* The free radicals, formed when unstable polyunsaturated vegetable oils and spreads are oxidised, attack and damage healthy body cells. The body's defence system is alerted and white blood cells are released causing inflammation. Cell damage can lead to conditions such as heart disease, Type 2 diabetes and cancer.

2. *Inflammation.* The low fat diet has resulted in a high intake of carbohydrate. Refined and processed carbohydrates such as bread, breakfast cereals, polished rice, potato, snack food and sugar-sweetened beverages has resulted in blood glucose spikes and surges of the weight-promoting hormone insulin. This, along with the high intake of pro-inflammatory polyunsaturated *omega-6* vegetable oils and spreads, has been another factor causing chronic inflammation in the body. Chronic inflammation is the precursor to many long-term conditions.

3. *Weight gain and insulin resistance.* The high carb/low fat diet stimulates insulin that increases insulin resistance, appetite and the storage of body fat. Insulin resistance stimulates the production of yet more insulin - and then it becomes a vicious cycle......until the person becomes obese and/or develops Type 2 diabetes.

4. *An abundance of triglycerides, small dense LDLs and shortfall of protective HDLs.* Carbohydrate that is not used for energy is stored in the liver and cells as a carb reserve called glycogen. However, when the stores are full, any further intake is converted into fat. This has been shown to increase blood triglyceride levels, fatty liver (non-alcoholic fatty-acid disease) and harmful small dense LDLs and reduce protective HDLs.

5. *Cardiovascular disease (CVD).* Cell damage, inflammation, weight gain, insulin resistance, high blood triglycerides, fatty liver, small dense LDLs and a lack of HDLs are all risk factors for CVD. All these risk factors may be caused by a high carb/low fat diet.

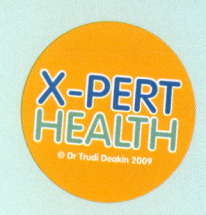

Focus on alcohol

Recommendations: The government advises that people should not regularly drink more than 3-4 units of alcohol a day for men (equivalent to a pint and a half of 4% beer) and 2-3 units for women (equivalent to a 175 ml glass of wine). 'Regularly' means drinking alcohol every day or most days of the week.

The more you drink above the safe limits, the more harmful alcohol is likely to be and it can lead to liver disease, pancreatitis, erectile dysfunction, high blood pressure, depression, damage to nerve tissue, cancer, obesity and addiction.

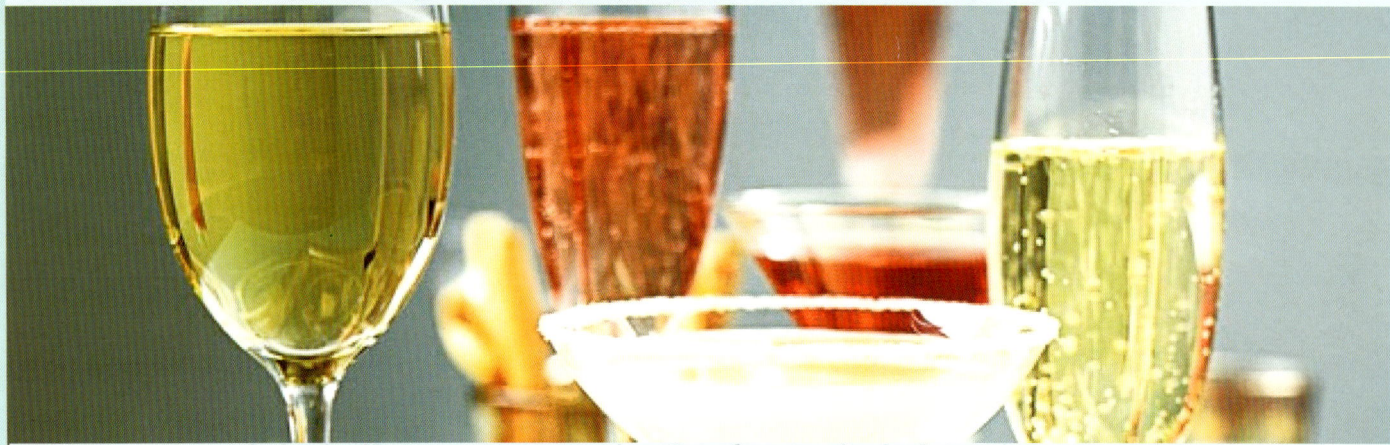

What is a unit of alcohol? One unit is 10ml or 8g of pure alcohol. It takes an adult around 1 hour to eliminate one unit of alcohol from their bloodstream, although this varies from person to person.

Alcohol by volume (ABV): Alcohol content is also expressed as a percentage of the whole drink. Look on a bottle of wine or a can of lager and you'll see either a percentage, followed by the abbreviation "ABV", or sometimes just the word "vol". Wine that says "13 ABV" on its label contains 13% pure alcohol.

The alcoholic content in similar types of drinks varies a lot. Some beers are 3.5% but this varies and some brands can be 5% ABV, or even 6%. The same goes for wine where the ABV of stronger wines can exceed 14%. This means that just one pint of strong beer or a large glass of wine can contain more than three units of alcohol, the upper daily unit guideline limit.

Measures and glass sizes: Spirits used to be commonly served in 25ml measures, which are one unit of alcohol, many pubs and bars now serve 35ml or 50ml measures. Large wine glasses hold 250ml, which is one third of a bottle. It means there can be nearly three units or more in just one glass. So if you have just two or three drinks, you could easily consume a whole bottle of wine – and almost three times the government's daily alcohol unit guidelines – without even realising. Smaller glasses are usually 175ml and some pubs serve 125ml.

Strategies for drinking less:
- If you drink wine at home, opt for small 125ml glasses and don't fill to the brim.
- Try and pour your own drinks. If your host is constantly topping up your half-filled glass, it's hard to keep track of how much alcohol you are drinking.
- Drink spritzers if you like wine, or pints of shandy if you're a lager drinker. You'll still get a large drink, but one that contains less alcohol. To reduce carbohydrate load, use sugar-free mixers.
- Opt for half pints if you prefer higher strength beer or try lowering the strength. You may not notice the difference.
- Alternate alcoholic drinks with sugar-free soft drinks.
- If you are uncertain about how much you are drinking, ask the bar staff. Do they pour doubles or singles? How big is their glass of wine?

If you would like to calculate your weekly average, you may find it useful to visit the following website that provides an automated alcohol unit and calorie calculator: http://www.drinkaware.co.uk/understand-your-drinking/unit-calculator or use the smartphone version of the MyDrinkaware drink tracking tool. It's free and simple to use.

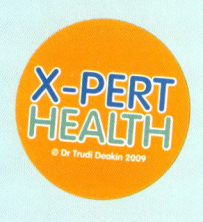

Focus on alcohol

The table below provides alcohol units, calorie and carbohydrate content for a range of drinks. The carbs are colour-coded green, amber & red for easy reckoning (N.B. As there is large variation between brands, use for general guidance only. Manufacturers also modify the nutritional values from time to time).

Drink	ABV	Units	Calories	Carbs
Red wine - small glass (125ml) e.g. Cote du Rhone, Chianti, Rioja, Shiraz, Merlot & Cabernet Sauvignon	12% to 14.5%	1.5 to 1.8	85-110 kcal	1g
White wine (dry) - small glass (125ml) e.g. Muscadet, Sancerre, Bianco Moncaro	12% to 12.5%	1.5 to 1.6	85-110 kcal	1g
White wine (medium) - small glass (125ml) e.g. Champagnes, Pinot Grigio, Sauvignon Blanc, Chablis, Chardonnay, Cava Brut	11.5% to 13.5%	1.5 to 1.7	85-110 kcal	3g
White wine (sweet) - small glass (125ml) e.g. Sauternes, Moscato	14.5%	1.8	150 kcal	12g
Rose wine - small glass (125ml) e.g. Stowells Light Shiraz, Blossom Hill, Jacob's Creek Shiraz*, Marques De Caceres Rosado	5.5% to 13.5%	0.7 to 1.7	70-126 kcal	1g*- 8g
Fortified wine - pub measure (50 ml) e.g. Port, Ruby, Sherry, Special Reserve, Vintage	17.5% to 20%	1	70-80 kcal	3-6g
Whisky - small measure (25ml) e.g. Highland Malt, Scotch, Irish, Bells	40%	1	55 kcal	0g
Brandy - small measure (25ml) e.g. Armagnac, Calvados	40%	1	55 kcal	0g
Gin & Vodka - small measure (25ml) e.g. Gordon, Hendrick's, Greenalls	37.5% to 40%	1	55 kcal	0g
Cider - 1 pint (568ml) Magners Strongbow	 4.5% 5%	 2.6 2.8	 210 kcal 244 kcal	 16g 22g
Alcopops - 275ml bottle e.g. Smirnoff Ice, WKD	4%	1.1	184 kcal	31g
Lager - 1 pint (568ml) 0% e.g. Becks Blue, Holsten Alcohol Free 4% e.g. Fosters*, Carling, Stella Artois 5% e.g. Carlsberg Export, Kronenbourg*, Peroni, San Miguel, Bud bottle, Grolsch	 0% 4% 5%	 0 2.3 2.8	 100-140 kcal 170-190 kcal 200-255 kcal	 25 - 35g 10*- 15g 12*- 25g
Bitter - 1 pint (568ml) 3.6% e.g. Tetley 4% e.g. Boddingtons*, Wainwrights	 3.6% 4%	 2 2.3	 187 kcal 170-210 kcal	 19g 10*- 20g
Stout e.g. Guinness Draft	4.1%	2.3	210 kcal	20g

N.B. Serving sizes in the table above are for a small glass of wine (125ml) and a small shot of spirits (25ml) but be aware that pubs and restaurants may serve 175ml glasses of wine and 35ml of spirits as their standard measure. Ciders and ales in the table above are for a 1 pint serving and therefore if 1/2 pint servings are consumed, the units, calories and carbs need to be halved.

www.xperthealth.org.uk

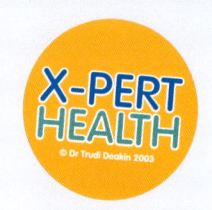

Zero and low calorie sweeteners

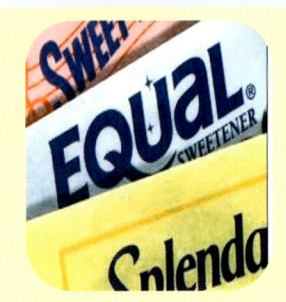

Zero and low calorie sweeteners reduce calories and carbohydrate load and can replace sugar in drinks and baking.

Be aware that when zero and low calorie sweetener are mixed with bulking agents for use in baking, the bulking agent is maltodextrin, which is basically glucose. However, one tablespoon of the sweetener (2.5g) only weighs one-tenth of sugar (25g) but does the same job. **Top tip:** use a tablespoon to measure the sweetener rather than weighing scales or it will result in a product that is too sweet with an aftertaste, cost you a fortune and contain far too many carbs.

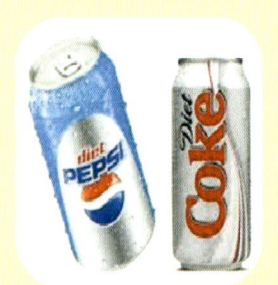

Sweeteners currently available in the UK are listed below:

1. Artificial Sweeteners

Acesulfame-K (the "K" refers to the mineral potassium) is a commonly used table top sweetener that has 200 times the level of sweetness as sugar. It is also a common additive to chewing gum, jam, dairy products, frozen desserts, drinks and baked goods. It is not broken down, nor is it stored in the body. After being consumed, it is quickly absorbed and then rapidly excreted through the kidneys, unchanged. Acceptable daily intake: 9mg per kg of body weight. Brand examples: Canderel and Silver Spoon Sweetener.

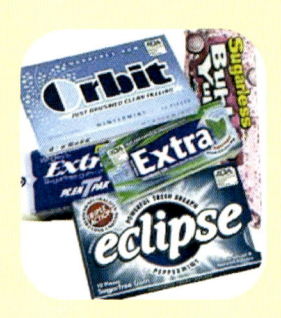

Advantages
- It does not affect blood-glucose levels
- No calories
- It can be used in cooking and baking
- It is approved for use during pregnancy

Disadvantages
- It can leave a bitter aftertaste
- Animal studies have indicated higher use to be associated with greater risk of cancers. However, these claims have been dismissed by the European Food Safety Authority (EFSA)

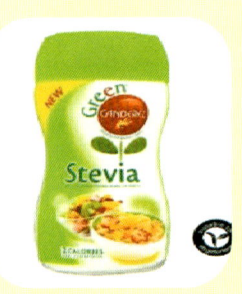

Aspartame

Aspartame is one of the most popular artificial sweeteners. It is derived from a combination of two amino acids: phenylalanine and aspartic acid to produce a substance that is 180-200 times sweeter than sugar. Acceptable daily intake: 50mg per kg of body weight. Brand examples: Canderel and Silver Spoon Sweetener.

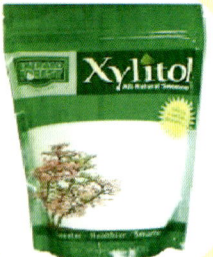

Advantages
- It adds very little or no calories to foods and drinks as only a tiny amount is required to create the sweetness of sugar
- Appears safe for pregnant women

Disadvantages
- Aspartame cannot be used for baking or cooking as it is not stable in heat or for long periods in liquid form
- Aspartame has been subject to more scare stories than any other sweetener, ranging from allergies and premature births to liver damage and cancer. The European Food Safety Authority (EFSA) conducted a comprehensive review of the evidence in 2013 and concluded that aspartame was safe for human consumption, including pregnant women and children.

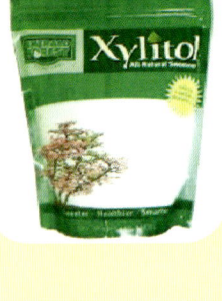

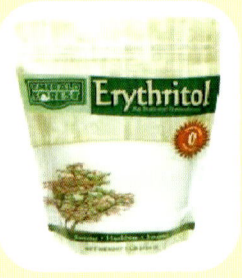

www.xperthealth.org.uk

Zero and low calorie sweeteners

Saccharin

Saccharin is an organic molecule derived from petroleum. It is the oldest artificial sweetener. It is calorie-free and 300 to 400 times sweeter than sugar. Some people find it has a bitter or metallic aftertaste. A wide variety of foods and drinks have saccharin added to them, including baked goods, chewing gum, drinks and table top sweeteners. Saccharin is also used in cosmetic products (such as toothpaste, mouthwash and lip gloss), as well as vitamins and medications. It is not broken down when digested. It is slowly absorbed into the system and rapidly excreted, unchanged, by the kidneys. Acceptable daily intake: 5mg per kg body weight. Brand examples: Sweetex and Hermesetas.

Advantages

- Due to its potency, only minute quantities are needed
- Its sweetness isn't affected by heat

Disadvantages

- Animal studies indicate heavy usage of saccharin to be associated with bladder cancer. Human studies have yet to show a clear association but people in certain subgroups, such as heavy smoking males, may be at increased risk
- Women are advised to use saccharin carefully during pregnancy as the substance can cross the placenta

Sucralose

Sucralose is 600 times sweeter than sugar. It is usually mixed with the bulking agent, maltodextrin. This enables it to be used as a substitute for sugar in food recipes. Acceptable daily intake: 15mg per kg body weight. Brand examples: Splenda.

Advantages

- Sucralose is calorie-free, is not considered a carbohydrate by the body, and has no effect on blood glucose levels
- It can be used as a baking ingredient and doesn't lose its sweetness with heat (N.B. do not weigh, use a tablespoon to measure)
- It is not thought to have a bitter aftertaste
- Sucralose has no effect on tooth decay and is commonly found in oral health products, such as chewing gum

Disadvantages

- The bulking agents used can add around 12 calories and 3g carbs per tablespoon which are usually not listed on the packaging
- The use of sucralose can change the texture in baking recipes and can also add an 'artificial' taste
- There are claims that studies in rats have linked the use of sucralose to organ damage and reduce levels of beneficial bacteria within the gut. However, in a review of the evidence, the EU's Scientific Committee on Food concluded that sucralose is safe for human consumption, is not harmful to the immune system, does not cause cancer, infertility, pose a risk to pregnancy or affect blood glucose levels

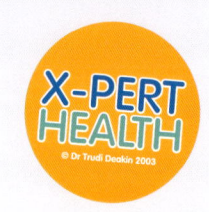

Zero and low calorie sweeteners

2. Natural sweeteners

Stevia

Derived from a plant in South America, it has been used for centuries by native Indians in Paraguay. Stevia is a calorie-free herb that is used as a replacement for sugar and artificial sweeteners. Marketed as a "natural sweetener", manufacturers market steviol glycosides to consumers looking for a healthier alternative to sugar. It is sold as a herbal powdered extract and is incredibly sweet being 200-300 times the sweetness of sugar. Acceptable daily intake: 4mg per kg body weight. Brand examples: Stevia and Truvia.

Advantages

- Stevia is classed as an all-natural herbal product
- It has been thoroughly tested around the world and found to be completely non-toxic
- It does not raise blood glucose levels. Although it is absorbed by the body it is rapidly eliminated in faeces and urine
- It is extremely heat stable and can be used in cooking and baking

Disadvantages

- Stevia does not caramelise as sugar does
- The granulated version contains maltodextrin, which contributes carbohydrate if eaten in large quantities
- Studies conducted by US researchers in the 1980s suggested that DNA changes occurred when stevia was tested with a certain bacteria. However it was approved by the EU in 2010 after the European Food Safety Authority (EFSA) carried out a comprehensive analysis of all the available evidence and concluded it was safe for human consumption
- It can give an unpleasant aftertaste

Sugar alcohols (polyols)

Erythritol, mannitol, xylitol and sorbitol are found in plant foods such as fruits and berries, and are also available as sweeteners. Whilst digested slowly, polyols are not fully absorbed into the body and can therefore cause diarrhoea in some people if consumed in large amounts.

Advantages

- About 60 times sweeter than sugar with fewer calories (per gram: sugar 4kcal, erythritol 0.2kcal, mannitol 1.5kcal, xylitol 2.4kcal, sorbitol 2.5kcal)
- Has a clean, cool pleasant taste
- No effect on tooth decay
- Beneficial for people on a low carb diet as polyols have very little impact on blood glucose and have been shown to have other beneficial influences on metabolic health

Disadvantages

- Consuming certain amounts of the sugar alcohols can cause some people to experience a laxative effect. Acceptable daily intake: none specified.

N.B. Erythritol is recommended as it is almost calorie free, has a pleasant taste, provides no side effects in the majority of people and is an excellent sugar substitute when baking.

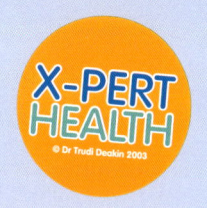

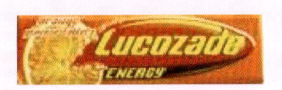

Glycaemic index

Carbohydrate Food

HIGH GI (quick-releasing)
- Glucose / Lucozade
- Cornflakes / Rice Krispies
- Cheerios / Coco Pops
- Puffed Wheat / Rice cakes
- French bread / Crumpets
- Plain biscuits e.g. Morning Coffee
- Potatoes (baked/mashed/chips)
- Crispbread / Crackers

MEDIUM GI
- Bread (white/wholemeal)
- Rice (white & brown)
- Oatmeal biscuits / Scones
- Ryvita / Basmati rice
- Pitta breads / Chapatti
- New & Sweet potatoes
- Sugar / Jam / Fizzy drinks
- Shredded Wheat / Weetabix
- Rich Tea & Digestive biscuits
- Crisps / Popcorn / Muffins
- Breads (granary/wholegrain)
- Fruit & Fibre / Special K cereal

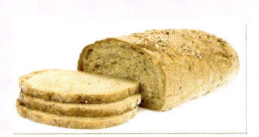

LOW GI (slow-releasing)
- Muesli / Porridge
- Sultana Bran / All-Bran
- Milk (cows/soya/almond)
- Fromage frais / Yoghurt
- Fruit / Vegetables
- Pulses (lentils/peas/beans)
- Fruit loaf / Dried fruit
- Tinned fruit / Fruit juice
- Chocolate / Ice cream / Custard
- Pasta (fresh/dried)
- Rye / Pumpernickel bread
- Baked beans / Dhal / Nuts

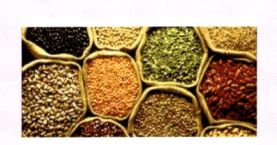

Glycaemic index (GI) is the rate that glucose from carbohydrate food impacts on blood glucose levels. Consuming glucose in isolation e.g. dextrose tablets or Lucozade impacts on blood glucose levels immediately and therefore glucose is given a GI ranking of 100. If foods release glucose quickly they are called HIGH GI foods with an index above 70 and those which break down slowly are called LOW GI foods with an index below 55.

Although the **amount** of carbs consumed is the most important factor for blood glucose control, the **type** of carbs should also be considered as low GI meals will cause a slower rise in blood glucose levels.

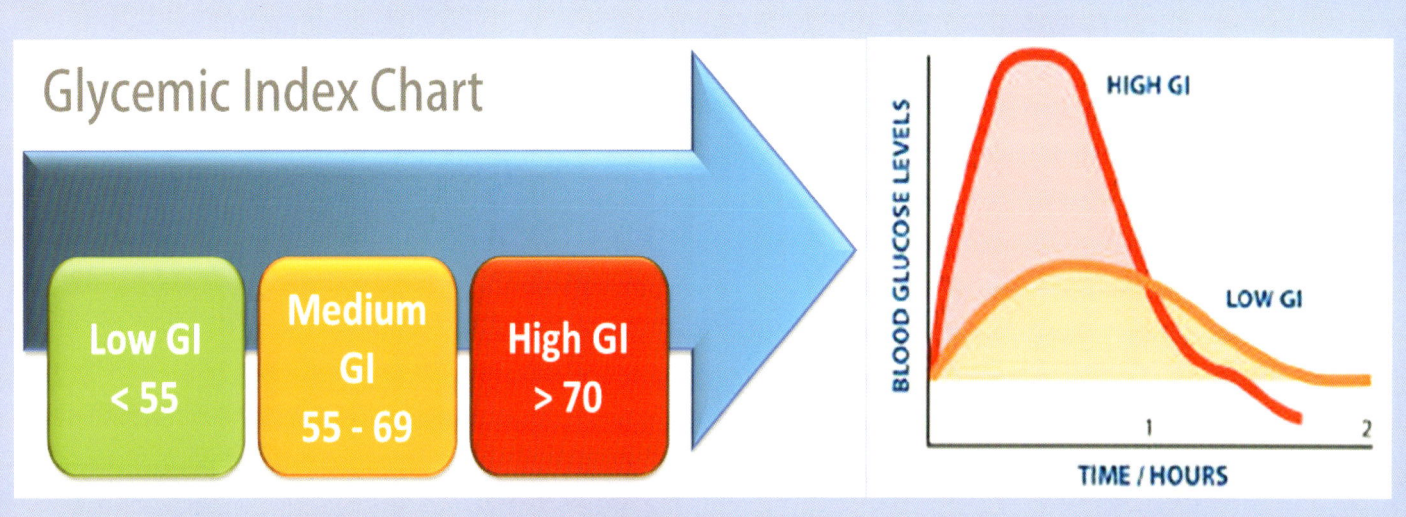

Glycemic Index Chart

- Low GI < 55
- Medium GI 55 - 69
- High GI > 70

www.xperthealth.org.uk

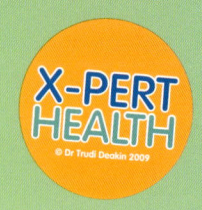

Reading and understanding food labels

Nutritional information on packaging can help you to understand what nutrients the food contains and allows you to compare different foods and brands.

1. The ingredients list

All ingredients have to be listed in order of the greatest weight. Therefore, in the example shown [pizza], the highest content is 'wheat flour' and lowest content 'black pepper'.

Individual ingredients can be listed under different names, for example, added sugars may be listed as sugar, sucrose, glucose, glucose syrup, invert syrup, maltose, fructose, lactose etc.

2. The nutritional information

A table will display the amount of each nutrient in that food. Some products will provide more information than others, including nutrients per serving, type of carbohydrate and the type of fat.

Many products display nutritional information *per 100g* and *per serving*. The amount *per serving* is useful if you eat the recommended serving size. The *per 100g* allows comparison with different products/brands. It also helps you identify whether a food or drink contains 'a lot' or 'a little' sugar, fat, saturates, fibre and salt by referring to food labelling guides. A Food Labelling Guide with a magnifying glass (so you can read the label!) may be purchased from the X-PERT online shop at www.xperthealth.org.uk.

Reference Intake of an average adult per day

Calories	2000 kcal
Total fat	70g
Saturates	20g
Total carbs	260g
Sugars	90g
Protein	50g
Salt	6g

3. Reference Intake (RI) Labelling

Reference Intakes [RIs] (previously known as Guideline Daily Amounts [GDAs]) are guidelines about the appropriate amount of particular nutrients and energy required for a healthy diet. Because individual requirements are different for all people, **RIs are not intended as targets and they are not all appropriate when following a low carb/high fat dietary approach** as the carb intake will be lower and fat intake higher.

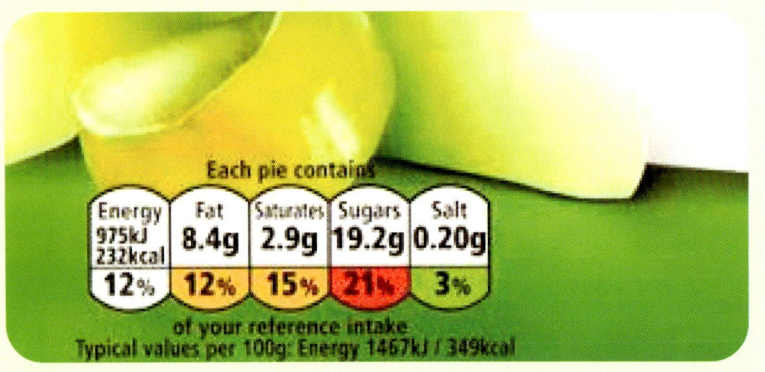

The RI labelling can be found on the front of some food packaging. It states the amount (g) and percentage (%) of calories, fat, saturates, sugar and salt per serving. However, limitations are: total carbs are not displayed on the front of packaging; the colour coding can be misleading for a low carb/high fat dietary approach.

Reading and understanding food labels

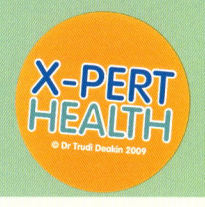

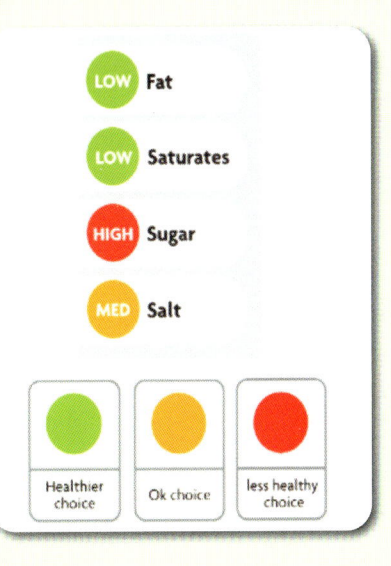

4. Traffic light labelling

Many foods have traffic light labelling to help consumers understand the amount and type of nutrients a product contains and how these compare to government recommendations. It also allows people to compare different products and brands.

The traffic light colours are used for fat, saturated fat, sugar and salt. Most foods are labelled with a mixture of the 3 colours and low fat eating guidelines encourage people to choose those with more green and amber lights and fewer red lights.

The table below identifies whether a food or drink is low in particular nutrients (green), medium (amber) or high (red) per 100g or per portion. **N.B. The guidance has been developed for a low fat diet and therefore if you adopt an alternative dietary approach the Traffic Light Labelling will not be applicable for fat and salt.**

Dietary approach guidance for food per 100g

	Low Fat, High Carb Diet	Mediterranean Diet	Low Carb, High Fat Diet
Carbs	To appetite	To appetite	Less than 10g per 100g
Sugars	Less than 5g per 100g	Less than 5g per 100g	Less than 5g per 100g
Fat	Less than 3g per 100g	To appetite	To appetite
Saturates	Less than 1.5g per 100g	Less than 1.5g per 100g	To appetite
Fibre	More than 3g per 100g	More than 3g per 100g	More than 3g per 100g
Salt	Less than 0.3g per 100g	Less than 0.3g per 100g	To taste

Number of portions should be adjusted for weight control

5. Confusing?

The reference intakes and traffic light guidance has been developed to help people follow a low fat, high carbohydrate diet. When adopting a low carb high fat lifestyle or a Mediterranean-style of eating it will be more helpful to use the guidance from the table on the right.

However, carbohydrate and fibre amounts will not be presented on *front of package* and you will have to read the nutritional table which is normally found on the *back of package*. The sample nutritional table (below right) informs the consumer that there are 18.2g carbs per serving (1 crumpet). Take note of the total carbohydrate not just the section that states "of which sugars" as sugar is only part of the carb content of a food product.

Some foods display a red traffic light but may be beneficial for health e.g. oily fish, cheese, nuts.

Pages 58 to 68 present the carbohydrate content of 160 foods and drinks. These are organised in food groups and the carbohydrate content calculated for a standard portion. The last two columns provide information to let you know if a food product is virtually carb free (green light), contains a small amount of carbs and therefore requires portion control (amber light) or is high in carbohydrate and therefore should be restricted or avoided (red light).

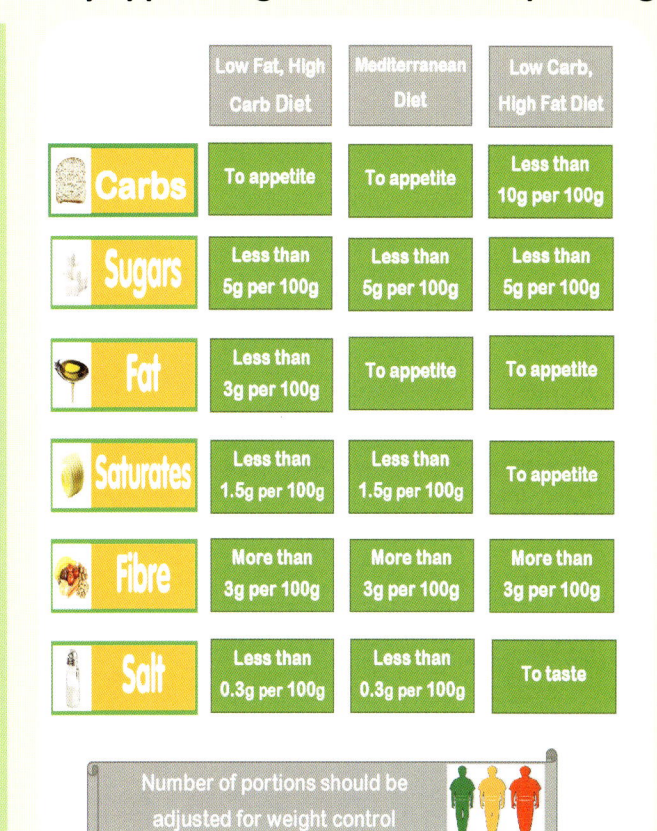

Back of package nutritional information

Nutrition Typical Values	per 100g	per crumpet (approx. 46g)		RI Average adult
Energy value (Calories)	820 kJ 195 kcal	380 kJ 90 kcal		2000 kcal
Fat	0.7 g	0.3 g	Low	70 g
(of which Saturates	0.2 g	0.1 g)	Low	20 g
Carbohydrate	39.5 g	18.2 g		260 g
(of which Sugars	3.9 g	1.8 g)	Low	90 g
Fibre	2.5 g	1.2 g		24 g
Protein	5.8 g	2.7 g		50 g
Salt	1.2 g	0.6 g	Med	6 g

RI = Reference Intake

www.xperthealth.org.uk

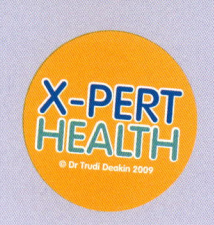

Carbohydrate awareness from food labels

Food/drink	Food image	Carb content per 100g	Portion size	Carbs per portion (g)	Low carb traffic light	Impact on blood glucose
Apples (1 small)		11.8	130g	15.3	Red	Large
Apple Juice (1 small glass)		10.3	150ml	15.5	Red	Large
Banana x 1 small (80g peeled / 128g with skin)		23.2	80g	18.5	Red	Large
Blueberries (4 heaped tablespoons)		6.9	80g	5.5	Amber	Medium
Broccoli (2-3 tablespoons)		1.8	80g	1.4	Green	Small
Carrots (2 tablespoons)		6.1	80g	4.9	Amber	Medium
Dried fruit (raisin & apricot - 1 dessert spoon)		67.2	25g	16.8	Red	Large
Grapes (approx. 12)		15.4	80g	12.3	Red	Large
Mandarin orange segments in juice (3 tablespoons)		8	80g	6	Amber	Medium
Mango (3-4 slices)		13.8	70g	9.7	Amber	Medium
Mediterranean roasted vegetables (2-3 tablespoons)		6.2	80g	5	Amber	Medium
Orange Juice (1 medium glass)		8.8	250ml	22	Red	Large
Peaches (in juice 2 tablespoons)		18	125g	14.5	Red	Large
Peas (mushy processed 2 tablespoons)		13.1	100g	13.1	Red	Large
Peas (frozen 2-3 tablespoons)		11	80g	9	Amber	Medium

= fruit & vegetables

Carb content

- 🟥 more than 10g per portion
- 🟧 2g to 10g per portion
- 🟩 less than 2g per portion

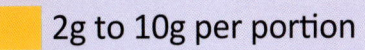

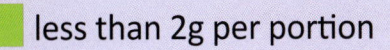

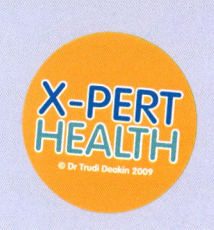

X-PERT HEALTH © Dr Trudi Deakin 2009

Food/drink	Food image	Carb content per 100g	Portion size	Carbs per portion (g)	Low carb traffic light	Impact on blood glucose
Soup - Carrot & Rocket Soup (1 bowl)		4.6	232g	10.7	🟥	Large
Soup - Vegetable cup soup (1 sachet)		5.5 (made up)	218ml	12 (made up)	🟥	Large
Strawberries (x7)		5.9	80g	4.7	🟧	Small
Sweetcorn (2 tablespoons)		16.9	80g	14	🟥	Large
Tomatoes (chopped - 1/2 can)		4	200g	8	🟧	Medium
Tomatoes (x1 raw)		3.1	80g	2.5	🟧	Medium
Bulgur Wheat (1/2 cup uncooked)		20.3	75g	15.2	🟥	Large
Bread - garlic (x 1/4 small baguette)		44	53g	23.3	🟥	Large
Bread - low carb mix (x1 slice of bread)		3.6	30g	1.1	🟩	Small
Bread - cinnamon & raisin bagel (x 1)		50.1	90g	45.1	🟥	Very Large
Bread - naan (x1)		46	90g	41.4	🟥	Very Large
Bread -pitta (x1)		47.9	60g	28.5	🟥	Large
Bread - seeded roll (x 1)		40.9	72g	29.4	🟥	Large
Bread - soya & linseed (x 1 slice)		27.3	33g	9	🟧	Medium
Bread - tortilla wrap (x 1)		50.2	62g	31.1	🟥	Very Large

🟩 = fruit & vegetables   🟨 = starchy carbs

www.xperthealth.org.uk

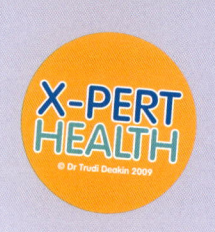

Carbohydrate awareness from food labels

Food/drink	Food image	Carb content per 100g	Portion size	Carbs per portion (g)	Low carb traffic light	Impact on blood glucose
Bread - white (1 slice)		36.4	37.8g	13.7	Red	Large
Bread - wholemeal (1 slice)		37.8	40g	15.1	Red	Large
Breadstick x 1		57.2	8g	4.6	Amber	Medium
Breakfast biscuits (x 1)		68	12.5	8.5	Amber	Medium
Cereal - brunch bar, raisin (x 1)		65	32g	21	Red	Large
Cereal - chocolatey squares (1 small bowl)		64.7	30g	19.4	Red	Large
Cereal - Cornflakes (1 small bowl)		84	30g	25	Red	Large
Cereal - porridge oats (3-4 tablespoons)		70.8	50g	35.4	Red	Very Large
Cereal - shredded wheat bitesize (small bowl)		68.7	40g	27.5	Red	Large
Cereal - Swiss style muesli (2 tablespoons)		62.5	45g	28.1	Red	Large
Cereal - wheat bisks (x 2)		69	37g	25.5	Red	Large
Chapatti (x1 small)		46.3	45g	20.8	Red	Large
Crispbread - mixed grain (x 1 cracker)		66.7	9.5g	6.3	Amber	Medium
Crumpet (x 1)		39.5	46g	18.2	Red	Large
Pasta - spaghetti (1/2 chilled packet, cooked)		29.7	280g	83.1	Red	Very Large

= starchy carbs

Carb content

- 🟥 more than 10g per portion
- 🟧 2g to 10g per portion
- 🟩 less than 2g per portion

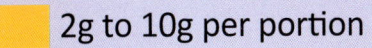

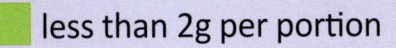

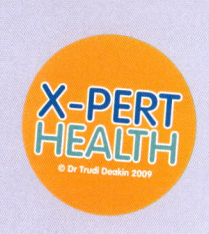

X-PERT HEALTH © Dr Trudi Deakin 2009

Food/drink	Food image	Carb content per 100g	Portion size	Carbs per portion (g)	Low carb traffic light	Impact on blood glucose
Pizza (1/2 pepperoni deep pan)		31	200g	62	🟥	Very Large
Pizza (1/2 thin crust cheese feast)		29.7	128g	38	🟥	Very Large
Potato (boiled x 3 egg-sized)		16.1	100g	16.1	🟥	Large
Potato (mashed 1/2 pack - 200g)		13.7	200g	27.4	🟥	Large
Potato (oven chips)		24	134g (cooked)	32	🟥	Very Large
Rice - Chinese style (x 1/2 pack)		27.1	140g	37.9	🟥	Very Large
Rice (1/2 microwave packet)		30.9	125g	38.6	🟥	Very Large
Rice Noodles (1/2 pack)		25.9	188g	48.6	🟥	Very Large
Biscuits - Chocolate Fingers (x 4 biscuits)		60	21g	12.6	🟥	Large
Biscuits - Rich Tea (x 2)		71.1	16.6g	11.8	🟥	Large
Biscuits - Digestives (x 2)		62.9	29.6g	18.6	🟥	Large
Biscuits - Twix (x 2 fingers)		64.6	50g	32.2	🟥	Very Large
Bombay Mix (small handful)		50	40g	20	🟥	Large
Cake - chocolate (x 1 very small slice)		53.5	64g	34	🟥	Very Large
Chocolate - Coffee Creams (x 2)		76.9	18g	14.2	🟥	Large

🟨 = starchy carbs   🟧 = sugary carbs

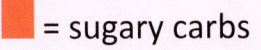

www.xperthealth.org.uk

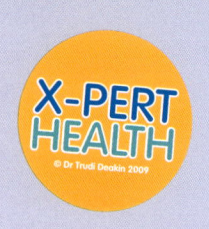

Carbohydrate awareness from food labels

Food/drink	Food image	Carb content per 100g	Portion size	Carbs per portion (g)	Low carb traffic light	Impact on blood glucose
Chocolate - Dairy Milk (4 chunks)		56.5	22.5g	12.5	Red	Large
Chocolate - dark 85% cocoa (3-6 squares)		26.4	20g	5.3	Amber	Medium
Chocolate - diabetic (6 squares)		49.7 (polyols 33.1)	25g	Available 4.1	Amber	Medium
Chocolate - Thornton's Classics (x 2)		64	26g	16.6	Red	Large
Crisps - Doritos (approx 1/2 66g pack)		55.4	30g	16.6	Red	Large
Crisps - 1 bag		52	30g	15.6	Red	Large
Crisps - Tyrrells (1/4 150g pack)		49	37.5g	18.4	Red	Large
Dessert - blackcurrant & madagascan vanilla (x1)		39.4	73g	28.7	Red	Large
Dessert - coconut milk with pineapple & chilli (x1)		21	100g	21	Red	Large
Dessert - strawberry trifle (1/4 pack)		17.4	150g	26.1	Red	Large
Fizzy Drink - Coca Cola (x 1 can)		10.6	330ml	35	Red	Very Large
Fizzy Drink - Diet Coca Cola (x 1 can)		0	330ml	0	Green	None
Fizzy Drink - Lucozade (x 1 bottle)		17.2	380ml	65.4	Red	Very Large
Fizzy Drink - sugar free (x 1 can)		0.6	500ml	3	Amber	Medium
Hot Chocolate Drink (x 1 sachet)		69.3	25g	17.3	Red	Large

■ = sugary carbs

Carb content

🟥 more than 10g per portion
🟧 2g to 10g per portion
🟩 less than 2g per portion

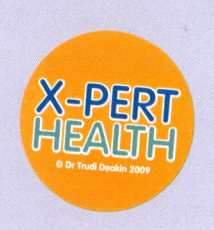

X-PERT HEALTH © Dr Trudi Deakin 2009

Food/drink	Food image	Carb content per 100g	Portion size	Carbs per portion (g)	Low carb traffic light	Impact on blood glucose
Ice Cream - Magnum Classic (x1)		29	79g	23	🟥	Large
Ice Cream - Magnum White (x1)		33	79g	26	🟥	Large
Ice Cream - Vanilla (x1 scoop)		23.2	55g	12.7	🟥	Large
Jaggery Goor - cane sugar (x 1 matchbox-size chunk)		95	30g	28.5	🟥	Large
Jam - reduced sugar (x 1 teaspoon)		43	15g	6.5	🟧	Medium
Jam - strawberry (x 1 teaspoon)		60.5	15g	9.1	🟧	Medium
Jelly - sugar-free (x 1 sachet)		15.6	23g sachet	0.4	🟩	Very Small
Sweetener - artificial (Splenda x 1 tsp)		97.7	0.5g	0.5	🟩	Very Small
Sweetener - polyol (xylitol or erythritol x 1 tsp)		100g (polyol)	1- 4g	1-4 (polyol)	🟩	Very Small
Sweets - Haribo (mini pack)		79	40g	31.6	🟥	Very Large
Sweets - Indian - Gulabjam (x 1 sweet)		48.1	83g	40	🟥	Very Large
Sweets - Liquorice Allsorts (x 4 sweets)		77.8	25g	19.5	🟥	Large
Tarts - Cherry Bakewell (x 1)		65.6	48g	31.2	🟥	Very Large
Benecol (1 bottle)		7.1	67.5g	4.8	🟧	Medium
Cheese - light cheese spread (1 portion)		6.5	17.5g	1.2	🟩	Small

🟧 = sugary carbs 🟦 = milk & dairy

www.xperthealth.org.uk

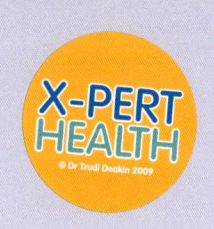

Carbohydrate awareness from food labels

Food/drink	Food image	Carb content per 100g	Portion size	Carbs per portion (g)	Low carb traffic light	Impact on blood glucose
Cheese - mature cheddar (matchbox size chunk)		0.1	30g	0	Green	None
Cheese - Philadelphia soft cheese (x1 dessert spoon)		5.1	30g	1.5	Green	Small
Cheese - reduced fat cheddar (matchbox size chunk)		3	25g	0.8	Green	Very Small
Cheese - Superlite (small matchbox size)		0.1	30g	0	Green	None
Custard - instant - just add water (1/3 packet made up)		16.8	26g powder	19	Red	Large
Milk - (1/3 pint)		4.8	200ml	9.6	Amber	Medium
Yogurt - fruit bio live organic (1 pot)		13.6	150g	20.4	Red	Large
Yogurt - Greek fruit (1 pot)		15.7	110g	17.3	Red	Large
Yogurt - Greek natural full fat (3 tablespoons)		4.9	150ml	7.4	Amber	Medium
Yogurt - Muller Light Strawberry fat free (x 1 pot)		7.8	175g	13.7	Red	Large
Butter (x 2 level teaspoons)		0.8	10g	0	Green	None
Cream - double (2 tablespoons)		1.6	30ml	0.5	Green	Very Small
Dips - various		5.6	133g	7.5	Amber	Medium
Margarine - Bertolli with butter (2 level teaspoons)		0.6	10g	0	Green	None
Margarine - Utterly Butterly (2 level teaspoons)		2.5	10g	0.3	Green	Very Small

■ = milk & dairy   ■ = fats

Carb content

- 🟥 more than 10g per portion
- 🟨 2g to 10g per portion
- 🟩 less than 2g per portion

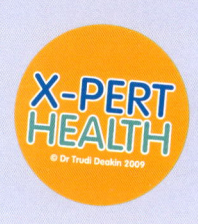

X-PERT HEALTH © Dr Trudi Deakin 2009

Food/drink	Food image	Carb content per 100g	Portion size	Carbs per portion (g)	Low carb traffic light	Impact on blood glucose
Mayonnaise - full fat (x 1 tablespoon)		0.2	14g	0	🟩	None
Oil - olive (x1 tablespoon)		0	15ml	0	🟩	None
Oil - sunflower (x1 tablespoon)		0	15ml	0	🟩	None
Oil - vegetable [rapeseed] (x1 tablespoon)		0	15ml	0	🟩	None
Bacon - back smoked (2 rashers)		0	70g	0	🟩	None
Baked Beans (x 1 one pot)		17.9	200g	35.8	🟥	Very Large
Beef Mince (lean, size of a deck of cards - uncooked)		0	100g (uncooked)	0	🟩	None
Beef Steak with Béarnaise Butter (x 1 steak)		0.2	150g (cooked)	0.3	🟩	Very Small
Cannellini Beans (x 2 tablespoons)		15.7	100g	15.7	🟥	Large
Chicken & Prosciutto in sauce (1/2 pack)		1.5	143g	2.2	🟨	Small
Chicken mini fillets in gravy (1 pack)		8.1	400g	32.4	🟥	Very Large
Chicken Yakitori (4 skewers)		7.8	100g	7.8	🟨	Medium
Curry - Pau Bhaji ready meal (x 1/2 pack)		9.3	150g	14	🟥	Large
Quorn - Peppered Steaks (x 1)		5.7	98g	5.5	🟨	Medium
Veggie burger x 1		17.5	120g	21	🟥	Large

🟧 = fats   🟦 = proteins (meat, fish & alternatives)

www.xperthealth.org.uk

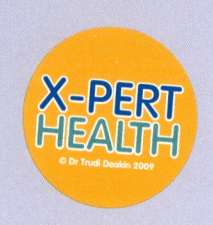

Carbohydrate awareness from food labels

Food/drink	Food image	Carb content per 100g	Portion size	Carbs per portion (g)	Low carb traffic light	Impact on blood glucose
Eggs - Scotch (x 1)		17.5	113g	19.8	Red	Large
Eggs - hen (x 1)		0	80g	0	Green	None
Fish - breaded haddock (x 1 fillet)		28	125g	35	Red	Very Large
Gammon Steak (x 1)		0	225g	0	Green	None
Ham (x 1 slice)		2	50g	1	Green	Small
Houmous (1 tablespoon)		15g	60g	9	Amber	Medium
Lentils - dried red split (2 tablespoons uncooked)		56.3	50g (uncooked)	28.2	Red	High
Mackerel (1 can)		0	110g	0	Green	None
Mackerel (1 smoked fillet)		0	145g	0	Green	None
Nuts - almonds (small handful)		6.9	25g	1.7	Green	Small
Nuts - salted peanuts (small handful)		10.9	25g	2.7	Amber	Medium
Pork loin (x 1 fillet)		0	175g	0	Green	None
Prawns (1/2 pack)		0	83g	0	Green	None
Prawns - king (1/2 pack)		0.8	75g	0.6	Green	Very Small
Quiche - tomato & cheese (1/2 pack)		20.3	165	33.5	Red	Very Large

■ = proteins (meat, fish & alternatives)

Carb content

🟥 more than 10g per portion
🟧 2g to 10g per portion
🟩 less than 2g per portion

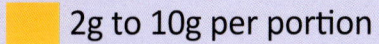

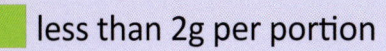

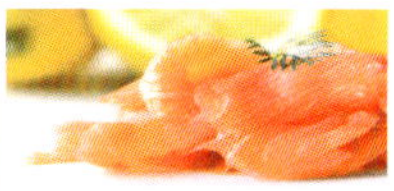

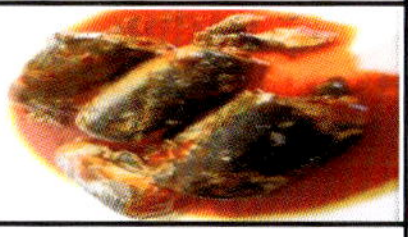

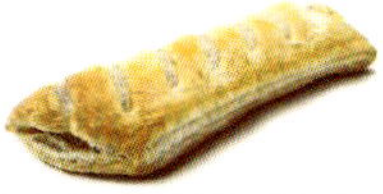

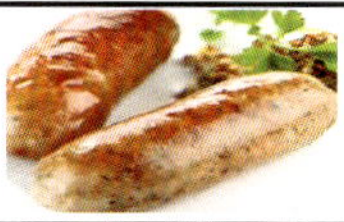

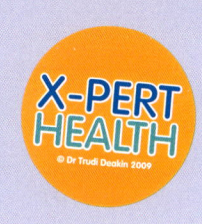

X-PERT HEALTH

Food/drink	Food image	Carb content per 100g	Portion size	Carbs per portion (g)	Low carb traffic light	Impact on blood glucose
Salmon - smoked (x 1 slice)		0.8g	35g	0.3	🟩	Very Small
Sardines in tomato sauce (x 1 95g can)		1.5	95g	1.4	🟩	Small
Sausage Roll (x 1 jumbo)		29.5	150g	44.3	🟥	Very Large
Sausages - bacon and cheddar (x 2)		5.1	84g	4.2	🟧	Medium
Sausages - Chorizo swirl sausage (x 1)	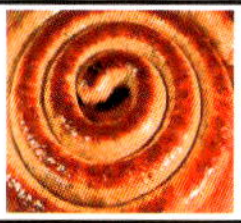	1.5	100g	1.5	🟩	Small
Sausages - high meat content pork (x 2)		0.5	133g	0.6	🟩	Very Small
Tuna (x1 160g can in brine - drained)		0	112g (drained)	0	🟩	None
Lager - Carling 4% (1 can)		2.2	500ml	11.2	🟥	Large
Lager - French Premium 4.8% (1 small bottle)		4.4	250ml	11	🟥	Large
Wine - Red 13% (1 small glass)		0.8	125 ml	1	🟩	Small
Cheese & Leek Chicken Gratin (1/2 pack)		2.8	170g	4.8	🟧	Medium
Chicken Arrabbiata (1 pack)		12.5	400g	50	🟥	Very Large
Cottage Pie (1 pack)		8.2	450g	36.9	🟥	Very Large
Indian meal - jalfrezi and tikka (1/2 pack)		22	595g	120	🟥	Very Large
Jerk chicken with rice & corn (1 pack)		9.6	380g	36.5	🟥	Very Large

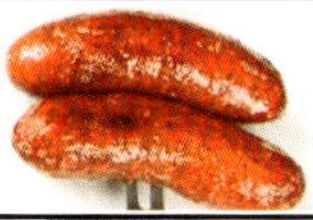

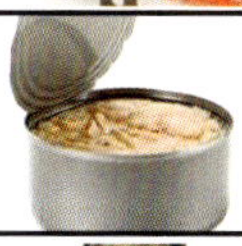

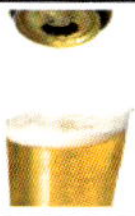

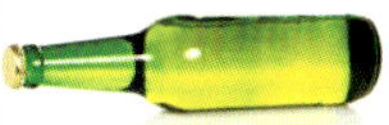

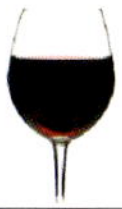

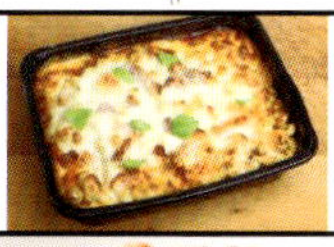

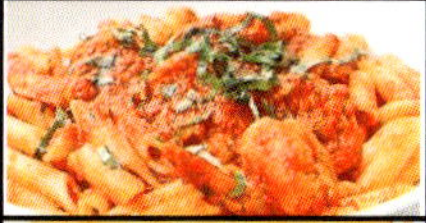

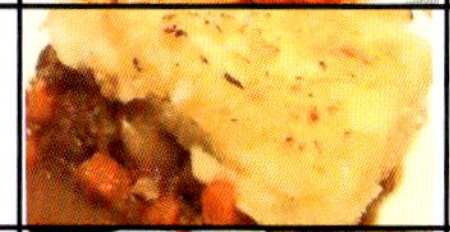

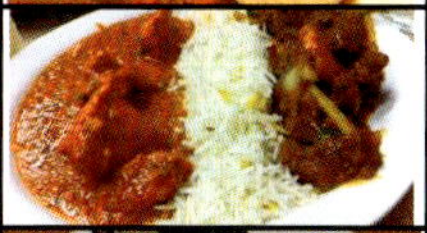

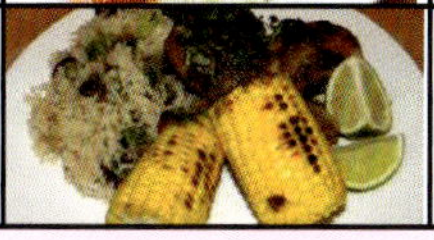

= proteins (meat, fish & alternatives)   = alcoholic drinks   = complete meals

www.xperthealth.org.uk

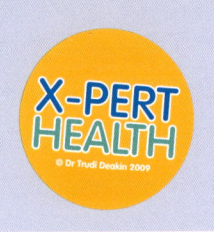

Carbohydrate awareness from food labels

Food/drink	Food image	Carb content per 100g	Portion size	Carbs per portion (g)	Low carb traffic light	Impact on blood glucose
Lasagne - beef (x 1 pack)		10.7	400g	42.8	🟥	Very Large
Pie - steak & ale (x 1)		23	200g	46	🟥	Very Large
Quorn - Cottage Pie (1/2 pack)		10	250g	25	🟥	Large
Chicken & Veg Casserole (1 pack)		9.9	440g	43.6	🟥	Very Large
Chicken Hotpot (1 pack)		10.5	320g	33.6	🟥	Very Large
Roast pork loin with apple & cider sauce (1 pack)		7.6	390g	29.6	🟥	Large
Salmon with potatoes, vegetables & sauce (1 pack)		7.8	385g	30	🟥	Large
Sandwich - tuna and sweetcorn (1 pack)		22.3	167g	37.2	🟥	Very Large
Spaghetti Carbonara (1 pack)		14.2	400g	56.8	🟥	Very Large
Spinach & ricotta cannelloni (1 pack)		14.9	400g	59.6	🟥	Very Large
Tomato & mozzarella tart (1/2 tart)		23.4	120g	28.1	🟥	Large
Vegetarian spicy three bean enchiladas (1/2 pack)		21.2	200g	42.4	🟥	Very Large
Fajita seasoning mix (1/8 pack)		41.5	3.75g	1.6	🟩	Small
Gravy granules (1/2 pint)		2.6 (as consumed)	20g = 1/2 pint	7.3	🟧	Medium
Sauce - tikka masala (1/2 pack)		11.7	185g	21.6	🟥	Large

⬜ = complete meals   🟪 = miscellaneous

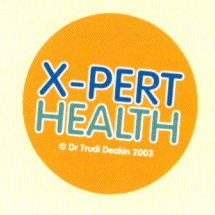

Suggested meal plans

To provide you with ideas of what to eat we have 7-day suggestions for breakfast, lunch, evening meal and snacks. Most people find that their appetite reduces when adopting a low carb high fat dietary approach and only eat 2 to 3 times per day.

The meal suggestions below are for you to mix and match according to your appetite. One day you may have breakfast, snack and evening meal and on another day you may have 1 snack and 1 meal. Experiment to see what works for you. Remember that old habits do take time to die and therefore if you are used to eating 3 meals plus snacks, it make take a few weeks to feel comfortable with your new eating pattern.

7-day breakfast ideas

Day 1	Day 2	Day 3	Day 4	Day 5	Day 6	Day 7
Bacon eggs sausages* fried mushroom 1/2 fried tomato butter (for frying)	Scrambled eggs made with butter & a variety of additions such as cheese, onion, peppers & fish	Fried kippers or mackerel with tomato	Walnut scone with butter (see recipe)	Berries with full fat Greek yogurt or cream	Omelette with a variety of fillings	Bacon sandwich with low carb bread (see recipe for English muffin)

*high meat content

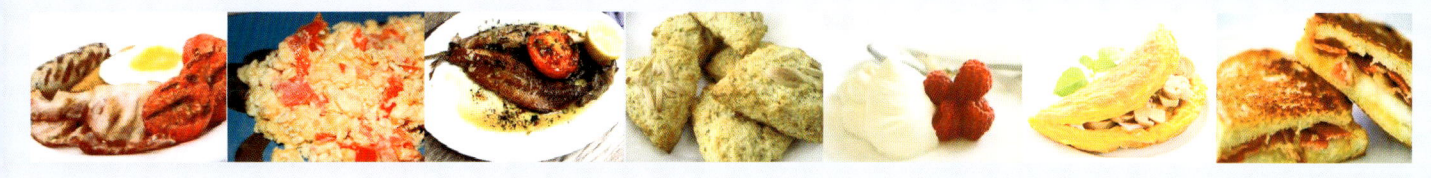

Snacks and desserts

Day 1	Day 2	Day 3	Day 4	Day 5	Day 6	Day 7
Hard Cheese	Full fat natural Greek yogurt	Dark bitter chocolate (70 - 100% cocoa solids)	Low carb biscuits (see recipe)	Pork scratchings	Full fat soft cheese with celery	Low carb dessert (see recipes)
Olives	Low carb cake (see recipe)	Nuts	Cold meat	Cucumber with full fat sour cream	Diabetic chocolate	Smoked salmon

www.xperthealth.org.uk

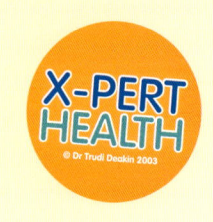

Suggested meal plans

Lunches

Day 1	Day 2	Day 3	Day 4	Day 5	Day 6	Day 7
Homemade soup	Cold meat or fish with salad	Low carb pizza (see recipe)	Avocado and prawns with full fat mayo	Frittata with salad (see recipe)	Fish or chicken goujons with carrot chips (see recipes)	Homemade beef or mozzarella burgers with salad

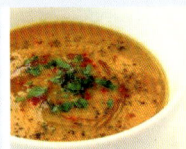

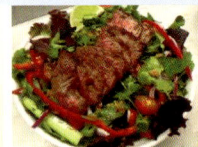

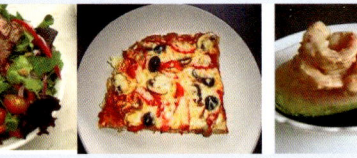

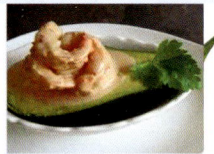

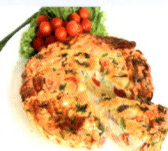

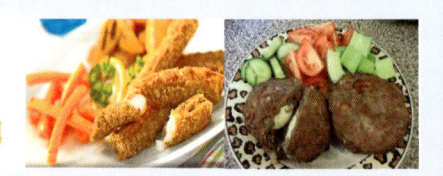

Evening meal

Day 1	Day 2	Day 3	Day 4	Day 5	Day 6	Day 7
Stir-fry with meat or fish	Chicken stuffed with cream cheese and wrapped in bacon (see recipe)	Steak with cauliflower mash (see recipe) and green beans	Lasagne with leek pasta (see recipe) and salad	Pork in cream and mushroom sauce served with courgette spaghetti (see recipe)	Steak & kidney almond crust pie with carrot, swede or celeriac fries (see recipes)	Chicken curry with cauliflower rice (see recipes)

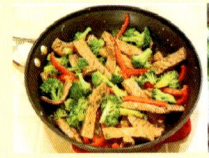

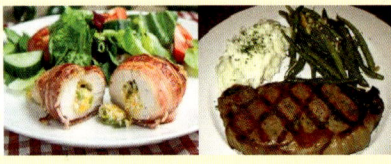

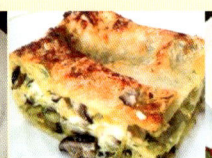

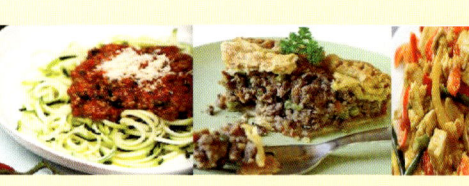

www.xperthealth.org.uk

Advert

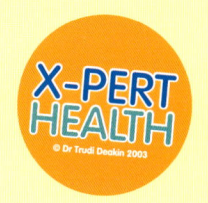

THE NATURAL LOW CARB STORE

Going low carb or ketogenic low carb doesn't need to mean deprivation or compromise, nor sacrificing yourself to artificial ingredients and sweeteners.

At the Natural Low Carb Store you can find everything you need for the ultimate low carb lifestyle... Why not try our luxury breakfast granolas or brilliant low carb almond porridge at only 5 grams of carbs per portion?

If Breakfast is not your thing we have amazing nut bars which are only 3 grams of carbs per bar and available in two great super food flavours.

With the Natural Low Carb Store you can even welcome back tasty chocolate treats, puddings and cakes knowing, with confidence, that they are low in carbs and free from artificial sweeteners. Our amazing Chefs have also developed delicious ready meals which are easy to prepare giving great variety and flavour to your low carb diet.

Use the code **XPERT15** to get **15% off** your first order and become a savvy low carber, living your low carb lifestyle the natural and sustainable way.

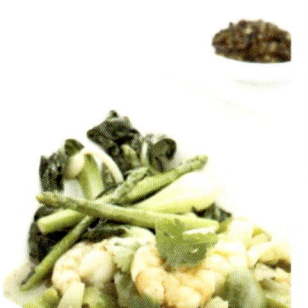

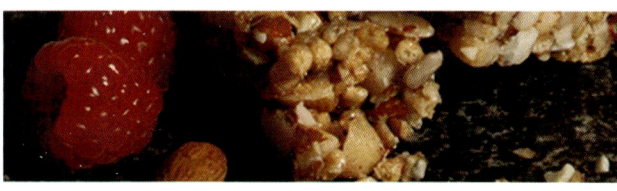

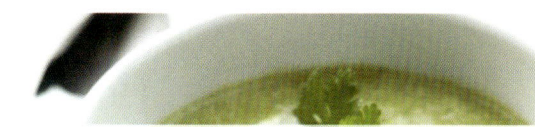

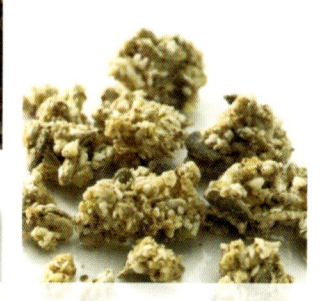

TRY OUR PRODUCTS TODAY AT WWW.NLCS.CO.UK

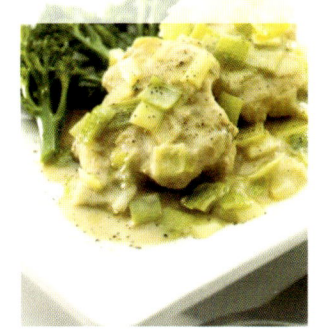

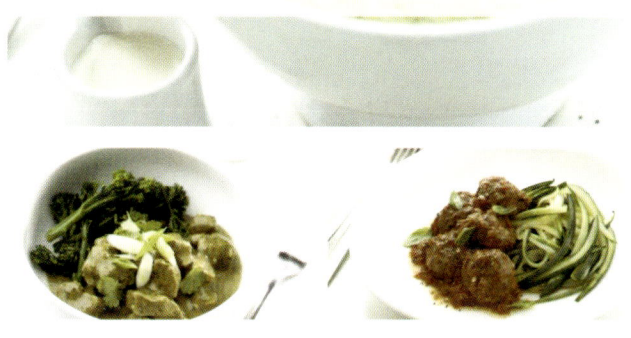

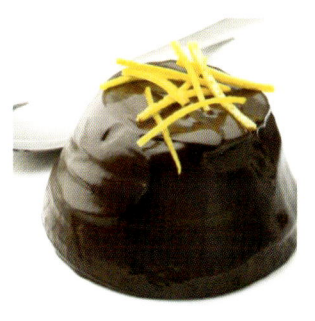

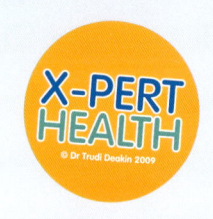

Low carb recipes

English muffin (low carb bread - 2 min microwave)
1 egg
1 tablespoon water
1 tablespoon extra-virgin olive or coconut oil
1 heaped tablespoon (30g) ground almonds
1 heaped tablespoon (20g) milled golden flax seed
¾ teaspoon baking powder
1 pinch sea salt
Optional: 1 teaspoon of seeds such as chia seeds

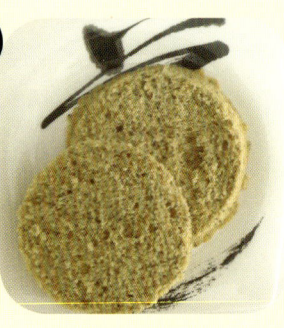

1 (86g) serving:
Per Serving
349 kcal
2.6g carbohydrate
6.8g fibre
32g fat
4g saturated fat
230mg sodium

1. In a small bowl, whisk egg with olive oil and water.
2. Whisk in remaining ingredients.
3. Microwave on high for two minutes or until the muffin feels firm to the touch.
4. Leave to cool.
5. Slice horizontally, toast or fill with your favourite ingredients.

Low carb thin & crispy pizza
200g mozzarella cheese, shredded
100g cheddar cheese, grated
3 eggs
1 teaspoon garlic powder
1 teaspoon dried basil, optional
Toppings: 75g pepperoni, 75g salami, 100g mushrooms, 100g green peppers (sauté in frying pan), 200g passata, 100g mozzarella cheese

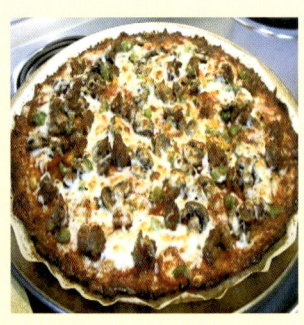

4 servings:
Per 271g Serving
534 kcal
8g carbohydrate
1g fibre
38g fat
19g saturated fat
1183mg sodium

1. Mix the cheeses, eggs, garlic powder and basil well.
2. Either grease a 16-inch pizza pan or line with greaseproof paper/nonstick foil.
3. Evenly spread the cheese mixture in the pan, almost to the edge, making it as thin as possible.
4. Bake at 200°C for 15-20 minutes until golden brown.
5. Spread passata, toppings and cheese. Keeping the oven rack in the center position, put the pizza under the grill until the cheese melted and bubbly, about 4-5 minutes.

N.B. Add variety by adding different toppings each time you make it.

Ground almond & walnut scones
250g ground almonds
2 teaspoons baking powder
100g walnut or pecan pieces
50g butter
50g mascarpone or full fat natural Greek yogurt
2 tablespoons zero/low calorie sweetener*
Pinch of salt

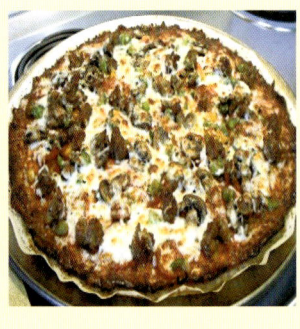

10 servings:
Per 51g Serving
252 kcal
3g carbohydrate
4g fibre
23g fat
4g saturated fat
50mg sodium

1. Mix the dry ingredients.
2. Melt the butter and add to dry ingredients.
3. Mix into a dough and portion into 10 scones.
4. Place on a baking tray and cook in a moderately hot oven (180°C) for approximately 20 minutes until set and golden brown.

N.B. the recipe can be adapted by omitting the mascarpone/yogurt and adding more butter instead, adding a small amount of cocoa powder to make chocolate scones or adding 25g psyllium husk powder to increase the fibre content. *e.g. Erythritol, Truvia, Stevia, Xylitol

Low carb recipes

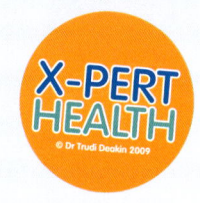

Almond & parmesan chicken/fish goujons

500g raw chicken/fish fillets (cut into strips)
50g grated parmesan cheese
50g ground almonds
1 or 2 eggs
Salt & pepper to taste, spices optional
Lard for frying

4 servings:
Per 185g Serving
446 kcal
2g carbohydrate
2g fibre
27g fat
9g saturated fat
323mg Sodium

1. Whisk eggs together in a bowl.
2. Mix the parmesan and ground almonds in another bowl. Add spices such as chilli if you wish.
3. Take a chicken/fish strip and dunk it in the egg mix.
4. Shake off any excess and drop it into the 'coating mixture'. Roll it around until fully coated and set it on a plate to set for 10 minutes. Repeat until all strips are coated.
5. Melt the lard* in either a deep frying pan or deep fat fryer and fry for 8 to 15 minutes until the chicken/fish is cooked and golden and crispy on the outside.

*Lard is an excellent fat for frying. It contains a healthy balance of monounsaturated and saturated fat (~50/50) and is stable to heat preventing oxidation and free radical production.

N.B. The coating mixture can be used to coat other foods such as prawns, mushrooms, mozzarella balls etc.

Spicy carrot french fries

6 fresh carrots
1 tablespoon ground black pepper
1 tablespoon red cayenne pepper
Lard for deep frying
salt to taste

4 servings:
Per 110g Serving
181 kcal
8g carbohydrate
3g fibre
15g fat
6g saturated fat
103mg sodium

1. Preheat lard in deep fryer or frying pan to 185°C.
2. Cut carrots into the size of French fries and place in bowl with peppers.
3. Mix to coat carrots on all sides.
4. Deep fry carrots in batches about 5 minutes until crispy brown and remove carrots to drain.
5. Salt to taste.

N.B. Omit the pepper if you do not want the carrot fries to be spicy. You could also use peeled swede or celeriac instead of carrots.

Spinach frittata

500g spinach leaves, chopped
2 tablespoons extra-virgin olive oil
1 medium onion, chopped
1 large clove garlic, minced
9 large eggs
2 tablespoons cream
50g grated parmesan cheese
2 tablespoons sun-dried tomatoes, chopped
Salt and freshly ground pepper to taste
80g goats cheese

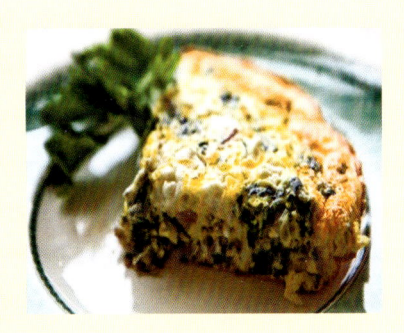

4 servings:
Per 318g Serving
412 kcal
6g carbohydrate
2g fibre
29g fat
12g saturated fat
442mg sodium

1. Preheat oven to 200°C. In a mixing bowl, whisk together eggs, cream and parmesan cheese. Add chopped sun-dried tomatoes and sprinkle with salt and pepper. Set aside.
2. Sauté onions and garlic in olive oil in an oven-proof, non-stick frying pan, until translucent. Add the chopped spinach and cook for a further 2-3 minutes.
3. Spread out spinach mixture evenly on bottom of frying pan. Pour egg mixture over spinach mixture. Use a spatula to lift up the spinach mixture to let egg mixture flow underneath.
4. Sprinkle bits of goats cheese over the top of the frittata mixture. When the mixture is about half set, put the whole pan in the oven. Bake for 13-15 minutes, until frittata is puffy and golden.

www.xperthealth.org.uk

Low carb recipes

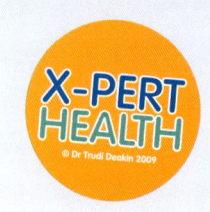

Chicken & cream cheese wrapped in bacon
4 boneless chicken fillets
150g Boursin garlic & herb full fat soft cheese
4 slices of bacon (or parma ham)
20g butter
Salt & pepper to taste

4 servings:
Per Serving
319 kcal
3g carbohydrate
15g fibre
32g fat
9g saturated fat
170mg sodium

1. Preheat the oven to 200°C.
2. Between 2 sheets of wax paper with a kitchen mallet or rolling pin flatten chicken breasts to 1.5 cm thickness.
3. Spread one-quarter of cream cheese over each chicken breast. Then dot with butter and sprinkle with salt.
4. Wrap up and secure with a toothpick. Then take one of the slices of bacon and wrap around chicken. Secure with another toothpick.
5. Bake uncovered for 35-40 minutes until juices run clear and the bacon is crispy.

Beef lasagne with leek pasta
2 large (600g) leeks
50g butter
1 onion, chopped
2 garlic cloves, crushed
3 peppers, chopped
150g mushrooms, chopped
500g minced beef
150ml red wine
200ml beef stock, made with 1 beef stock cube
200g can chopped tomatoes
2 tablespoons tomato purée
1 teaspoon dried oregano, 2 bay leaves, salt & pepper
2 tubs (400g) full fat soft cheese
50g extra-mature cheddar, grated
25g parmesan, finely grated

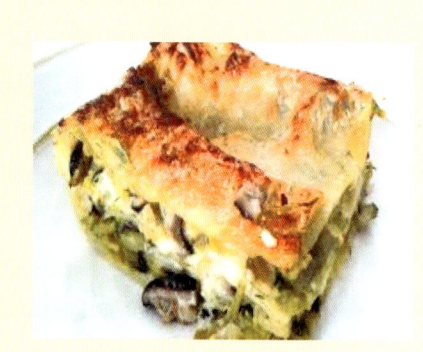

6 servings:
Per 382g Serving
558 kcal
16g carbohydrate
3g fibre
36g fat
9g saturated fat
710mg sodium

1. Trim the leeks until they are the same width as the lasagne dish. Cut the leeks lengthways.
2. Open out the leeks and remove the narrow leaves from the centre of each leek. Separate the larger leaves – these will become your 'lasagne'.
3. Fry the garlic & onion in butter in a large non-stick frying pan and then add the minced beef.
4. Stir in the chopped peppers and mushrooms and cook for a further 5 minutes.
5. Stir in the red wine and beef stock. Add the canned tomatoes, tomato purée, dried oregano, bay leaves into the pan and bring it to a simmer for 30 minutes. Season with black pepper.
6. Half fill a large saucepan with water and bring to the boil. Add the leek 'lasagne' and bring the water back to the boil. Cook the leeks for five minutes or until very tender.
7. Drain in a colander under running water until cold. Drain on kitchen paper or a clean tea towel.
8. Spoon a third of the mince mixture into a 2.5 litre lasagne dish. Top with a layer of blanched leeks. Repeat the layers twice more, finishing with leeks.
9. Place the soft cheese in a pan and melt over a lower heat. Add the cheddar cheese and bring to a simmer and cook for five minutes, stirring regularly until the sauce is smooth and thick.
10. Pour the cheese sauce over the leeks* and sprinkle the parmesan cheese over the top. Bake in preheated oven 200°C/Gas 6 for 30 minutes or until golden-brown and bubbling. Serve with a freshly dressed green salad. *You may wish to add a little cheese sauce between layers.

Low carb recipes

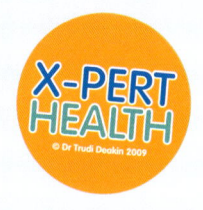

Steak and kidney pie with almond crust

For the filling
50g butter
700g stewing beef, diced
200g lamb kidney, diced
2 medium onions, diced
850ml beef stock
Salt and freshly ground black pepper, to taste
1 tablespoon Worcestershire sauce
15g cornflour (mixed to a paste with cold water)
For the crust
200g ground almonds / 50g coconut oil or butter (melted) / pinch of salt / beaten egg for glazing

8 servings:
Per 296g Serving
460 kcal
6g carbohydrate
4g fibre
30g fat
12g saturated fat
562mg sodium

1. Make the pastry by melting the coconut oil or butter, add the ground almonds and salt and mix together to form a dough. Refrigerate for about 30 minutes.
2. Heat the butter in a large frying pan, and brown the beef all over. Set aside, then brown the kidneys on both sides in the same pan. Add the onions and cook for 3-4 minutes.
3. Return the beef to the pan and add the stock and cornflour paste, stir well whilst bringing to the boil. Turn the heat down and simmer for 1½ hours without a lid.
4. Remove from the heat. Add salt, pepper and Worcestershire sauce and allow to cool completely. Place the cooked meat mixture into a pie dish.
5. Roll out the pastry (between 2 sheets of cling film) to the pie dish size and 5mm/¼in thick.
6. Using a rolling pin, lift the pastry and place it over the top of the pie dish. Trim and crimp the edges with your fingers and thumb.
7. Brush the surface with the beaten egg mixture and bake for 30-40 minutes in a preheated oven 200°C/Gas 6 until golden-brown. Serve with creamy cauliflower mash and steamed vegetables.

Cauliflower mash

900g cauliflower, trimmed
Sea salt (to taste)
60ml double cream (or to taste)
60g butter (or to taste)
30g grated parmesan cheese (optional)
60g cream cheese (optional)

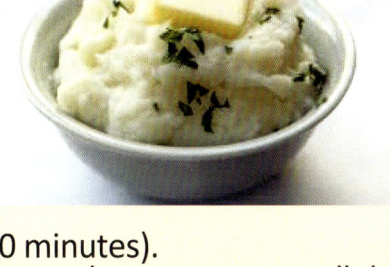

6 servings:
Per 185g Serving
195 kcal
5g carbohydrate
4g fibre
17g fat
10g saturated fat
249mg sodium

1. Chop the cauliflower including the core and add to a large pan of salted boiling water. Cook until completely tender (20-30 minutes).
2. Drain the cauliflower in a colander and press down to remove all the water.
3. Transfer the cauliflower to a food processor. Add the cream and puree until completely smooth.
4. Return to the pan. Re-heat when ready to serve adding the butter and cheese (if desired).

You can also make low carb mash using carrots, swede, parsnip or celeriac and can adapt the recipe by seasoning with fresh or roasted garlic, mustard or pesto.

Courgette spaghetti

4 courgettes
25g butter
10ml extra-virgin olive oil
1 clove garlic (crushed)
Salt & pepper to taste

4 servings:
Per Serving
98 kcal
5g carbohydrate
2g fibre
8g fat
4g saturated fat
153mg sodium

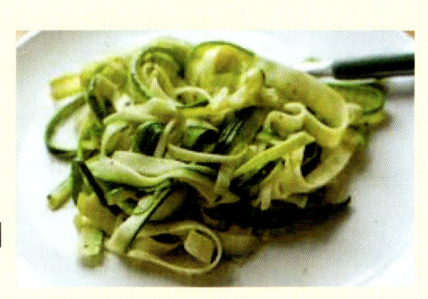

1. Really simple to make. You do not need a spiraliser unless you want even strips.
2. Wash, dry, top and tail the courgettes.
3. Use a potato peeler to peel strips. Work until you hit seeds and turn the courgette over and work on the other side.
4. Using a cook's knife cut into strips as evenly as you can manage and to your preferred thickness.
5. Heat the butter, olive oil and garlic gently. Add courgette and toss around for about 4 minutes. Add some freshly ground pepper and a pinch of sea salt.

www.xperthealth.org.uk

Low carb recipes

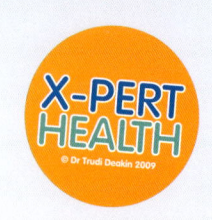

Chicken curry

4 chicken breasts, diced
1 onion, sliced
1 green/red pepper, sliced
1 large stalk of celery, sliced
1 teaspoon ground turmeric
1 teaspoon curry powder
1 teaspoon ground ginger
1 tablespoon plain or coconut flour
1 clove garlic, crushed
1 pint chicken stock
60g crème fraiche or double cream

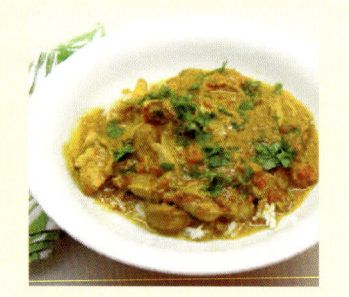

4 servings:
Per 420g Serving
476 kcal
6g carbohydrate
2g fibre
20g fat
4g saturated fat
670mg sodium

1. Fry the chicken breast until browned, add in the onion, green pepper, celery and garlic and cook for 10 minutes until soft. Add in the spices and flour and cook for a further 2 minutes.
2. Add in the chicken stock and stir thoroughly, simmer for 20-30 minutes.
3. Take off the heat and stir in the crème fraiche/cream. Serve with cauliflower rice or salad.

Cauliflower rice

900g cauliflower, trimmed
60g butter
2 cloves of garlic (crushed)
1 teaspoon sea salt
2 spring onions, thinly sliced
Freshly ground black pepper

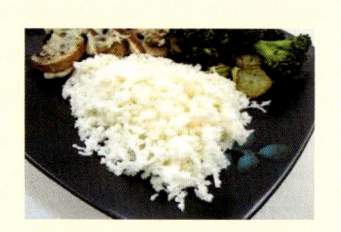

4 servings:
Per 170g Serving
114 kcal
5g carbohydrate
4g fibre
8g fat
5g saturated fat
572mg sodium

1. Grate the cauliflower, including the core, using medium holes of a grater (hand or food processor). Squeeze out as much water as possible.
2. Melt the butter in a large frying pan over medium heat. Add the garlic and sauté until the garlic sizzles.
3. Add the grated cauliflower, sprinkle with salt and stir-fry until tender crisp about 5-8 minutes.
4. Stir in the spring onions and season to taste with pepper.

Cheesecake

Base 250g ground almonds
2 tablespoons zero or low calorie sweetener*
75g butter (chopped into small pieces)
Topping
500g cream cheese (full fat)
14g gelatine plus 3 tablespoons water
3 eggs
3 tablespoons zero or low calorie sweetener*
Rind and juice of large lemon
100ml double cream

*e.g. Erythritol, Truvia, Stevia, Xylitol

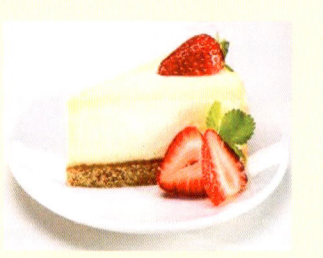

8 servings:
Per 115g Serving
374 kcal
3g carbohydrate
3g fibre
36g fat
17g saturated fat
190mg sodium

1. Rub the butter into the ground almonds, add the sweetener and mould into base of cake tin.
2. Bake in a pre-heated 200°C oven for around 10-15 minutes or until golden brown and crispy.
3. Separate eggs. Add sweetener and rind to yolks and beat. Add cream cheese and beat.
4. Soak gelatine in water for 5 minutes and then heat until dissolved (low heat – do not boil).
5. Add lemon juice to gelatine.
6. Add gelatine mix to cream cheese.
7. Lightly whip cream until just firm and stir in to cream cheese mix.
8. Beat egg whites until stiff and fold in to cream cheese mix.
9. Cover ground almond base with cream cheese mix and refrigerate until set.

Low carb recipes

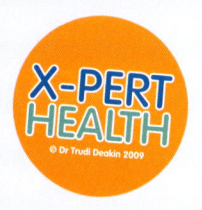

Chocolate Cake (3 minute microwave)
4 tablespoons ground almonds
1 tablespoon cocoa powder
¼ teaspoon baking powder
2 tablespoons zero or low calorie sweetener*
2 tablespoons butter, melted
1 tablespoon water
1 egg

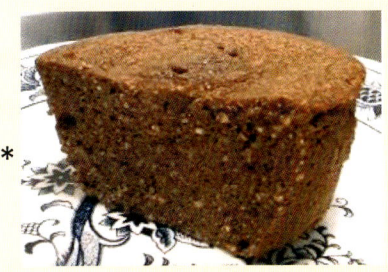

2 servings:
Per 169g Serving
209 kcal
2g carbohydrate
2g fibre
20g fat
9g saturated fat
114mg sodium

1. Mix the ground almonds, cocoa, baking powder and sweetener in a glass bowl.
2. Stir in the melted butter, water and egg. Mix well with a spoon or fork.
3. Scrape batter down evenly with a rubber spatula.
4. Microwave on HIGH 1 to 1½ minutes until set but still a little moist on top. Cool slightly and serve warm topped with whipped cream. N.B. 2 teaspoons coffee granules can be added instead of cocoa.

*e.g. Erythritol, Truvia, Stevia, Xylitol

Chocolate filled ginger biscuits
Biscuits: 200g ground almonds
2 tablespoons zero or low calorie sweetener*
1½ teaspoon ground ginger
1 teaspoon ground cinnamon
1 teaspoon baking powder
¼ teaspoon salt
2 teaspoons vanilla extract
1 large egg, lightly beaten
2 tablespoons butter, melted
Chocolate filling: 5 tablespoons butter
50g chocolate (80% cocoa)
2 tablespoons zero or low carb sweeteners*
25g cocoa powder & ¼ teaspoon vanilla extract

15 servings:
Per 35g Serving
156 kcal
4g carbohydrate
3g fibre
14g fat
5g saturated fat
83mg sodium

1. In a large bowl, whisk together ground almonds, sweetener, ginger, cinnamon, baking powder and salt. Stir in egg, melted butter, and vanilla and stir until dough comes together.
2. Roll out dough between two layers of parchment to ½ cm thickness. Cut into circles using a 5-cm diameter cookie cutter and place on lined baking sheet (you will get about 30 biscuits).
3. Bake for 15 minutes in preheated oven 150°C or until cookies are firm to the touch and just browning around the edges. Let cool in tray.
4. For the filling, melt butter, chocolate and sweetener together in a small saucepan over low heat. Stir in cocoa powder, vanilla and whisk until smooth. Remove from heat and let sit 5 to 10 minutes to thicken. Spread the underside of one cookie with chocolate filling and top with another cookie. Let set about 20 minutes.

*e.g. Erythritol, Truvia, Stevia, Xylitol

Ice cream
4 egg yolks
4 tablespoons zero or low calorie sweetener*
500ml double cream
1 teaspoon vanilla essence

6 servings:
Per 113g Serving
328 kcal
3g carbohydrate
0g fibre
34g fat
21g saturated fat
38mg sodium

1. Beat sweetener and egg yolks in a bowl with an electric mixer until pale and creamy.
2. In another bowl, whip cream until soft peaks form.
3. Gently fold sweetener and egg yolk mix into the cream.
4. Pour into a two-litre plastic container with a tight fitting lid and freeze overnight or until firm.

N.B. Cocoa or coffee could be added instead of vanilla essence. If using erythritol sweetener melt in a little boiling water first to prevent granulated texture.

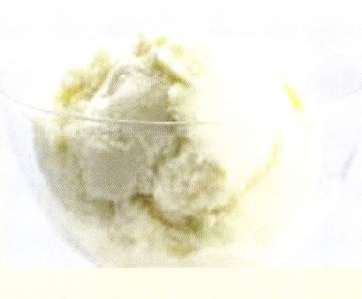

*e.g. Erythritol, Truvia, Stevia, Xylitol

www.xperthealth.org.uk

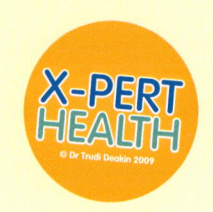

Where can I find products & information?

Products
1. Ketogenic Diet Resource http://www.ketogenic-diet-resource.com
2. Low carb bread mix - Sukrin Sunflower and Pumpkin Seed (available from Amazon)
3. Zero and low calorie sweeteners e.g. erythritol, xylitol, truvia and stevia (available from large supermarkets, health food shops & Amazon)
4. We hope to start stocking ingredients to support low carb cooking on our online shop at www.xperthealth.org.uk

Websites
1. Authority Nutrition http://authoritynutrition.com/low-carbohydrate-diets
2. Natural Ketosis http://www.naturalketosis.co.uk

Blogs
1. http://livinlavidalowcarb.com/blog/
2. http://alldayidreamaboutfood.com
3. http://peaceloveandlowcarb.com
4. http://www.ibreatheimhungry.com
5. http://lowcarblayla.blogspot.co.uk
6. http://247lowcarbdiner.blogspot.co.uk
7. http://carbwars.blogspot.co.uk

Facebook Page
Share your experiences, successes, challenges and recipes with others by visiting our Facebook page "X-PERT Health" or twitter @xperthealth

Books
1. Big Fat Lies by Hannah Sutter
2. The Art and Science of Low Carbohydrate Living and Low Carbohydrate Performance, both by J. Volek and S. Phinney
3. Carbs and Cals by Chris Cheyette and Yello Balolia
4. The Big Fat Surprise by Nina Teicholz
5. Grain Brain by David Perlmutter and Kristin Loberg
6. Keto Clarity by Jimmy Moore and Eric Westman
7. Nourishing Traditions by Sally Fallon and May Enig

Recipe Books
1. The Low Carb Gourmet by Karen Barnaby
2. The Low Carb High Fat Cookbook by Sten Sture Skaldeman
3. Low Carb Revolution: Comfort Eating for Good Health by Annie Bell

Analyse your own recipes
1. http://caloriecount.about.com/cc/recipe_analysis.php
2. http://www.myfitnesspal.com

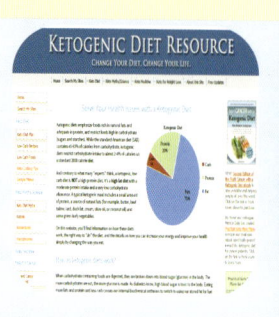

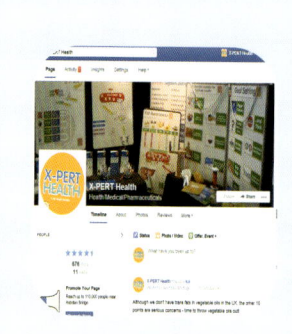

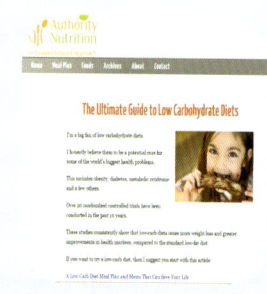

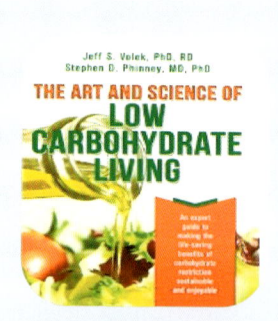

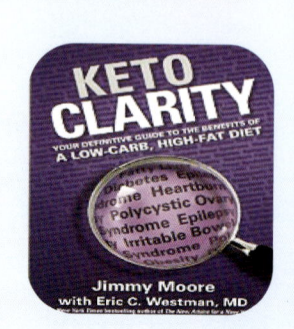

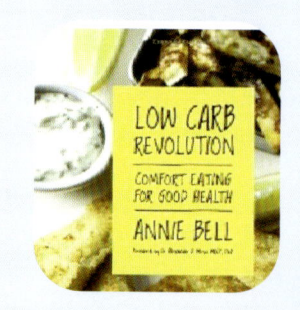

Health indicators

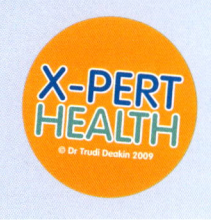

The monitoring health form (on page 88) lists the main health results that your care team (such as doctor, nurse, dietitian, pharmacist or specialist) takes into consideration when they monitor your health. If you know and understand what your health results are it may help you to self-manage your health. Ask for your results and complete the monitoring health form. Remember, the results are *your* health results!

If you have specific questions regarding your own health profile, write them down and discuss these with your healthcare team.

Health indicator	What does it mean?
Height (m)	Height is a measurement of how tall you are. It is usually measured in metres and centimetres.
Weight (Kg)	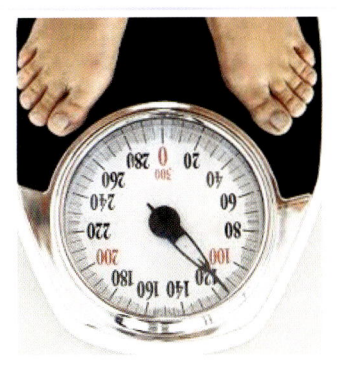 Weight is the measurement of your body weight in kilograms. If overweight, there are major health benefits from losing even a small amount of weight. Excess weight also makes it hard for your body to use insulin properly [insulin resistance] and therefore losing weight helps you to control blood glucose levels.
BMI (Kg/m^2) [weight for height calculation]	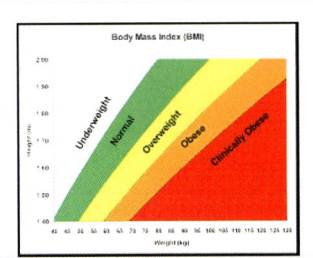 Body Mass Index [BMI] is an assessment of your weight for height and gives you an indication of whether you are underweight, normal weight, overweight or obese (see page 82).
Waist Size (cm)	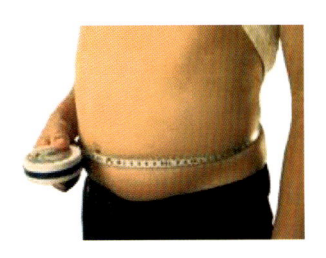 Waist size is a measurement midway between the lower rib and hip bone. If you gain weight around your middle, it will become harder to control blood glucose levels and it will increase your risk of developing heart disease.

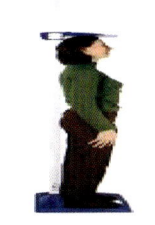

www.xperthealth.org.uk

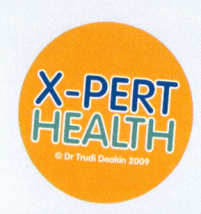

Health indicators

Investigation	What does it mean?
Blood Glucose (mmol/L)	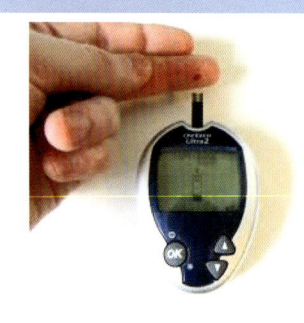 Blood glucose tests give an indication of the amount of glucose in the blood, but only at the time when the blood sample is taken. It involves pricking the finger, placing a drop of blood on a test strip for the meter to analyse. A fasting result can be taken after an overnight fast.
Glycated Haemoglobin "HbA1c" (mmol/mol)	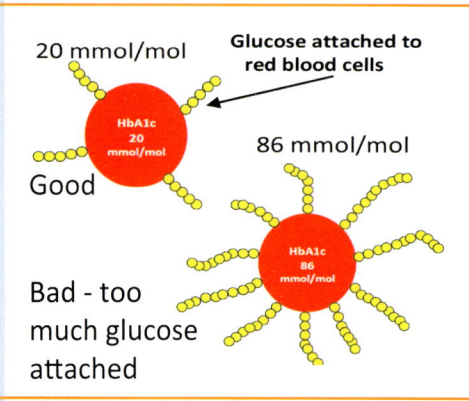 This blood test measures the amount of glucose that is being carried by the red blood cells in the body. It indicates the *average level of glucose in your blood over the last 2 to 3 months*. It is the most important tool to help people with diabetes understand how well their diabetes is controlled. A sample is taken from the vein in the arm and sent to a laboratory to be analysed.
Blood Pressure "BP" (mmHg)	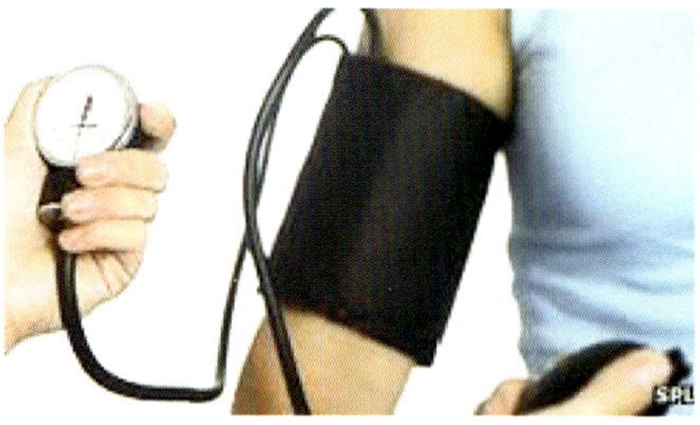 Blood pressure is the amount of force your blood exerts against the walls of your blood vessels. The first and larger number [systolic BP] is the pressure when the heart pumps the blood into the vessel. The second and smaller number [diastolic BP] is the pressure when the heart is at rest.
Total Cholesterol (mmol/L)	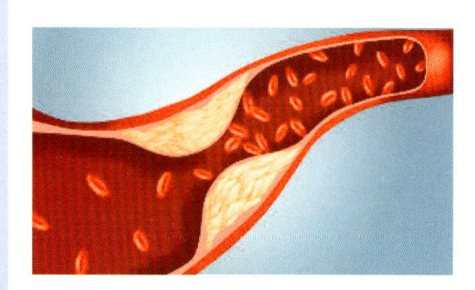 Cholesterol is a waxy substance that is essential to life. It is made in the body but small amounts are obtained from food. It is carried in the blood by carriers (lipoproteins) and if the levels of these carriers become unbalanced, the risk of heart disease increases.
HDL Particles (mmol/L) [cholesterol transporters]	HDL particles mop up any excess cholesterol in the body (roadsweeper) and carry it back to the liver where it is either excreted or recycled. It protects against heart disease. The levels increase when adopting a low carb high fat dietary approach.

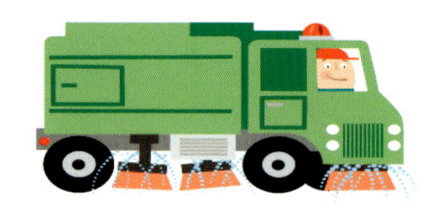

Health indicators

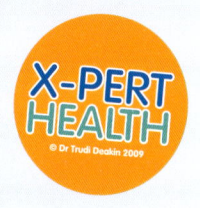

Investigation	What does it mean?
LDL Particles (mmol/L) [cholesterol transporters]	LDL particles are transporters (like trucks) that carry the essential cholesterol to where it is needed in the body. Eating carbs to excess causes these particles to shrink forming an abundance of small dense LDLs (cars) which damage the blood vessels causing the build-up of fatty deposits leading to heart disease and strokes.
Triglycerides (mmol/L)	Triglycerides is the fat we store in our body but we can also transport it in the blood. Raised blood levels increase risk of heart disease. Increased storage causes weight gain and fatty liver. Physical activity, eating oily fish, reducing carbs and alcohol and losing weight will help to lower levels.
Kidney Function Tests — Albumin to creatinine ratio [ACR]; Estimated glomerular filtration rate [eGRF]	The kidneys filter the blood, removing waste and water to make urine. Tests check how well the kidneys are functioning. The ACR test assesses whether too much protein is leaking into the urine and the eGFR test measures how much blood the kidneys are filtering.
Marker of inflammation: C-Reactive Protein (CRP)	A C-reactive protein (CRP) test is a blood test that measures the general levels of inflammation in your body. High levels are caused by infections but are also a risk factor for heart disease and Type 2 diabetes. Adopting a low carb high fat lifestyle has been shown to reduce CRP.
Liver function test: Gamma-glutamyl transpeptidase (GGT)	An enzyme found in the liver, GGT is used as a marker for liver disease or excessive alcohol intake. The test provides a very sensitive indicator of the presence of liver disease such as fatty liver. Fewer carbs means less glucose is available to be converted to fat.
Cardiovascular disease (CVD) 10-year risk score assessment QRISK2 — http://www.qrisk.org/	The QRISK2 CVD risk score assesses age, sex, ethnicity, smoking status, diabetes, family history, blood pressure, BMI, total cholesterol to HDL cholesterol ratio and other health conditions to calculate your risk of heart disease in the next 10 years.

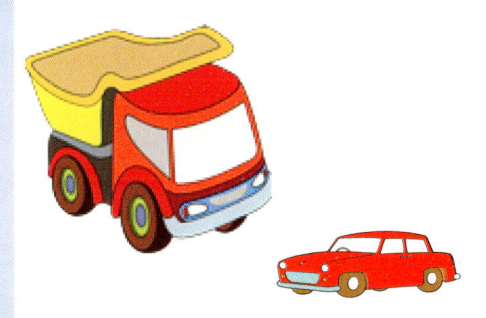

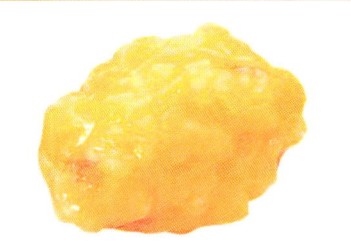

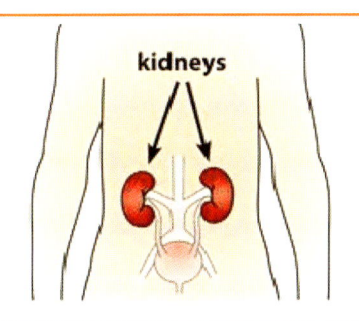

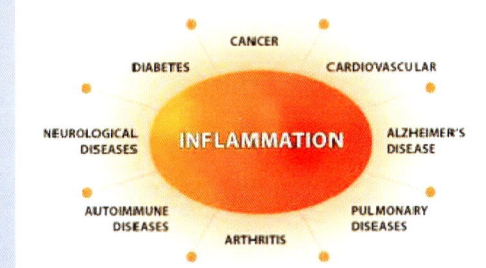

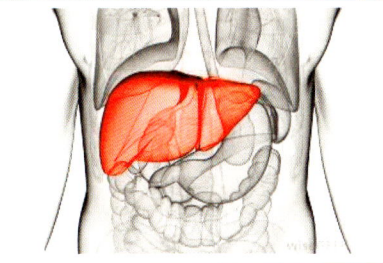

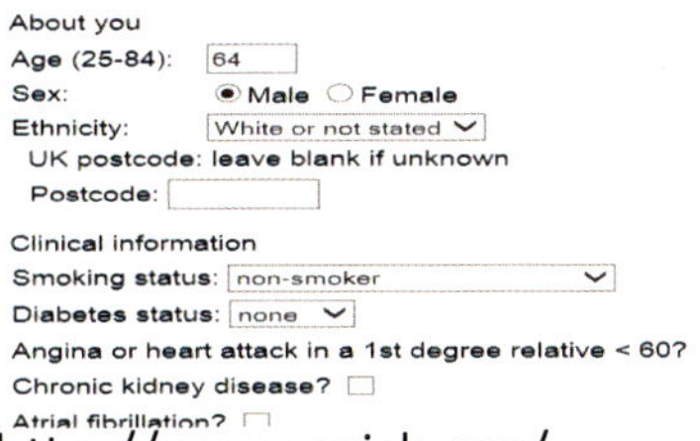

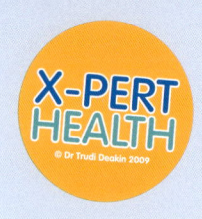

Health indicators

Are you a Healthy Weight?

Use the body mass index (BMI) chart below to check if you are a healthy weight. Find your height and draw a horizontal line across and then find your weight and draw a vertical line. Where the two lines meet will show you what weight section you are in. The World Health Organisation has published different BMI thresholds for Asian people as evidence suggests that people from black, Asian and other minority ethnic groups are at a higher risk of diabetes and other health conditions at a lower body mass index (BMI) than white populations.

WEIGHT lbs	100	105	110	115	120	125	130	135	140	145	150	155	160	165	170	175	180	185	190	195	200	205	210	215
kgs	45.5	47.7	50.0	52.3	54.5	56.8	59.1	61.4	63.6	65.9	68.2	70.5	72.7	75.0	77.3	79.5	81.8	84.1	86.4	88.6	90.9	93.2	95.5	97.7
HEIGHT in/cm	Underweight					Healthy						Overweight					Obese					Extremely obese		
5'0" - 152.4	19	20	21	22	23	24	25	26	27	28	29	30	31	32	33	34	35	36	37	38	39	40	41	42
5'1" - 154.9	18	19	20	21	22	23	24	25	26	27	28	29	30	31	32	33	34	35	36	36	37	38	39	40
5'2" - 157.4	18	19	20	21	22	22	23	24	25	26	27	28	29	30	31	32	33	33	34	35	36	37	38	39
5'3" - 160.0	17	18	19	20	21	22	23	24	24	25	26	27	28	29	30	31	32	32	33	34	35	36	37	38
5'4" - 162.5	17	18	18	19	20	21	22	23	24	24	25	26	27	28	29	30	31	31	32	33	34	35	36	37
5'5" - 165.1	16	17	18	19	20	20	21	22	23	24	25	25	26	27	28	29	30	30	31	32	33	34	35	35
5'6" - 167.6	16	17	17	18	19	20	21	21	22	23	24	25	25	26	27	28	29	29	30	31	32	33	34	34
5'7" - 170.1	15	16	17	18	18	19	20	21	22	22	23	24	25	25	26	27	28	29	29	30	31	32	33	33
5'8" - 172.7	15	16	16	17	18	19	19	20	21	22	22	23	24	25	25	26	27	28	28	29	30	31	32	32
5'9" - 175.2	14	15	16	17	17	18	19	20	20	21	22	22	23	24	25	25	26	27	28	28	29	30	31	31
5'10" - 177.8	14	15	15	16	17	18	18	19	20	20	21	22	23	23	24	25	25	26	27	28	28	29	30	30
5'11" - 180.3	14	14	15	16	16	17	18	18	19	20	21	21	22	23	23	24	25	25	26	27	28	28	29	30
6'0" - 182.8	13	14	14	15	16	17	17	18	19	19	20	21	21	22	23	23	24	25	25	26	27	27	28	29
6'1" - 185.4	13	13	14	15	15	16	17	17	18	19	19	20	21	21	22	23	23	24	25	25	26	27	27	28
6'2" - 187.9	12	13	14	14	15	16	16	17	18	18	19	19	20	21	21	22	23	23	24	25	25	26	27	27
6'3" - 190.5	12	13	13	14	15	15	16	16	17	18	18	19	20	20	21	21	22	23	23	24	25	25	26	26
6'4" - 193.0	12	12	13	14	14	15	15	16	17	17	18	18	19	20	20	21	22	22	23	23	24	25	25	26

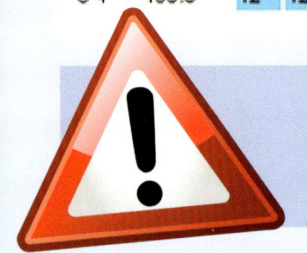

Note: The good news is that losing even a small amount of weight [between 5-10 kg] and keeping it off will help to keep blood glucose at normal levels.

Body Mass Index [BMI]

White/ Black People

Underweight	= less than 18.5 Kg/m^2
Healthy weight	= 18.5 to 24.9 Kg/m^2
Overweight	= 25 to 29.9 Kg/m^2
Obese	= 30 to 39.9 Kg/m^2
Very obese	= more than 40 Kg/m^2

South Asian People

Underweight	= less than 18.5 Kg/m^2
Healthy weight	= 18.5 to 22.9 Kg/m^2
Overweight	= 23 to 24.9 Kg/m^2
Obese	= 25 to 34.9 Kg/m^2
Very obese	= more than 35 Kg/m^2

Health indicators

Waist Measurements

Waist measurements are now considered to be a more accurate measure of future health risk than body weight.

Knowing your waist measurement is more useful than simply knowing if you are a healthy weight, overweight or obese.

The location of your body fat makes a difference to your risk of diabetes and heart disease. People with excess fat around their waist (so-called "apple" shape) have a greater risk of developing heart disease than people who carry weight on their hips and thighs (pear-shaped).

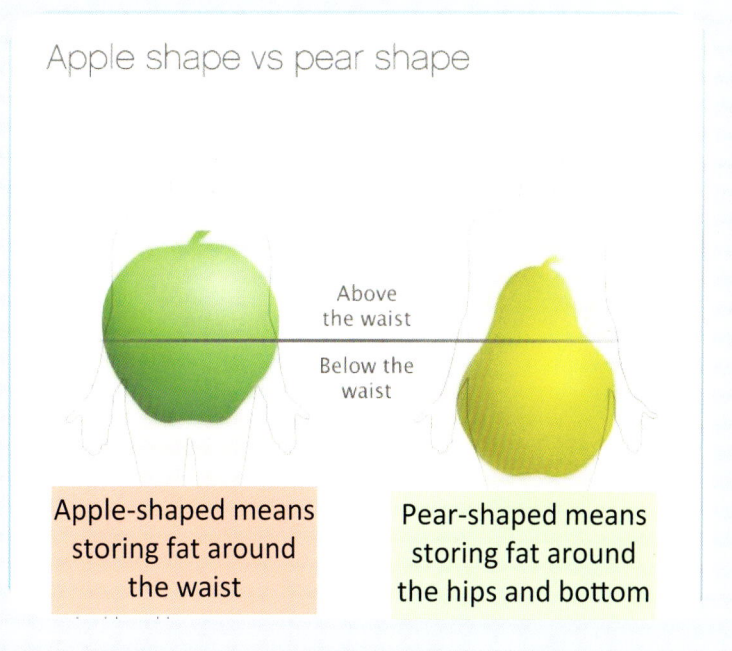

Apple shape vs pear shape

Apple-shaped means storing fat around the waist

Pear-shaped means storing fat around the hips and bottom

People who have excess abdominal fat and who are in the overweight category, may not realise that they have a greater health risk than people in the obese category who are not carrying excess abdominal fat.

How to measure your waist and assess your health risk

1. Take the measurement without clothes to provide a more accurate measurement.

2. Place a tape evenly around the middle point of your waist by doing the following:

    a. find the top of your hip bone (you could mark it with a pen);
    b. find the very bottom of your rib-cage (you could mark it with a pen);
    c. the half-way point between the two marks is the correct position of your waist;
    d. place the tape evenly around this point to measure your waist size;
    e. write down this number in centimetres (cm) to the nearest mm.

3. Try to be relaxed and breathe out gently when reading the measurement. Do not 'suck in' the stomach.

4. Ensure the tape is snug but does not push tightly into the skin.

5. Take the measurement twice to check the reading.

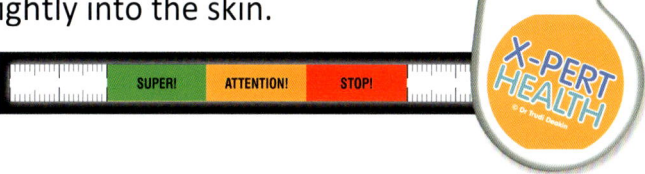

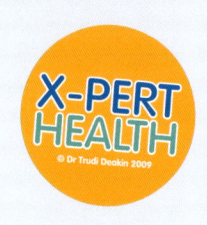

Waist measurements

Top tips: If you have difficulty feeling your rib-cage or hip bone or both, you may find it easier to place your hand, palm down, on your stomach. Place your middle finger on your tummy button and measure your waist just above your index finger.

If you have a prolapse, which has resulted in your tummy button falling below your waist, you may find it easier to slightly bend to the side and measure your waist at the indent.

Consistency is the key! It is therefore advisable to measure your own waist circumference and use the same technique on each occasion.

Remember:
1) Your waist is normally above the trouser line.
2) Breathe out whilst taking the measurement as breathing-in will give a false reading!

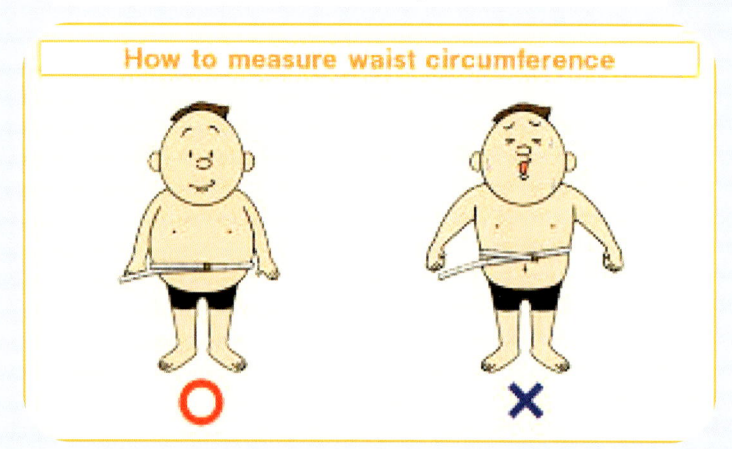

How to measure your waist

What does my waist measurement mean?

Fat around the abdomen is associated with increased risk of health problems. Use the guidance below to assess your risk

	Healthy Waist	Increased Risk	High Risk
For Men*	Less than 94cm (about 37 inches)	More than or equal to 94cm (about 37 inches)	More than or equal to 102cm (about 40 inches)
For Women	Less than 80cm (about 32 inches)	More than or equal to 80cm (about 32 inches)	More than or equal to 88cm (about 35 inches)

*For south Asian men the guidance is 90cm (35 inches) or less

Monitoring health

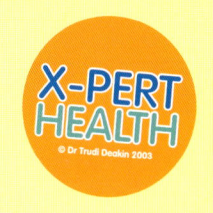

Date	Weight	Waist size	Blood glucose	Symptom relief

Monitoring health

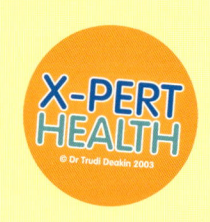

Date	Weight	Waist size	Blood glucose	Symptom relief

Monitoring health

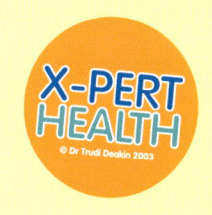

Overleaf (pages 88 -89) you can monitor the impact of a low carb high fat dietary approach on your health results. It is unlikely that all the health indicators listed will be tested by your healthcare team but some will be. At your next appointment ask your doctor or nurse what health indicators they monitor on a regular basis. Make sure that you obtain the results so that you can plot them in your handbook and compare the results over a period of time. For example, you may find that your blood pressure and/or triglyceride to HDL ratio reduces and/or your liver function improves. A simple explanation of common health indicators is available on pages 79 to 84.

We would love to hear about your experiences and would value you sending us a copy of any changes in your health results that have occurred due to the lifestyle over a period of time. You can either email them to admin@xperthealth.org.uk or mail to X-PERT Health, Linden Mill, Linden Road, Hebden Bridge, HX7 7DP.

Monitoring health

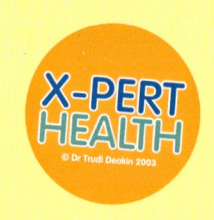

Health indicator	Reference range	Date:
Height (m)		
Weight (kg)		
Body Mass Index (BMI) (kg/m2)	🟩 18.5 to 24.9 = healthy 🟨 25 to 29.9 = overweight 🟥 More than 30 = obese	
Waist Size (cm) [M=male, F=female]	🟩 Healthy - less than: 94(M) 80 (F) 🟨 Increased risk: 94-102 (M) 80-88(F) 🟥 Greater risk - above:102 (M) 88 (F)	
Blood Glucose (mmol/l)	🟩 Fasting: below 6.0 🟩 Pre meal: below 5.9 🟩 2 hours post meal: below 7.8	
HbA1c (mmol/mol) [Average blood glucose]	🟩 20 to 41 (normal) 🟨 42 to 47 (pre diabetes) 🟥 48 and above (diabetes)	
Blood Pressure (mmHg)	🟩 Below 130/80 🟨 Below 140/90 🟥 Above 140/90	
Total Cholesterol (mmol/l)	No current recommendation Result used with other risk factors to assess CVD 10-year risk score (see below)	
HDL (mmol/l)	🟩 Men: 1.0 or above 🟩 Women: 1.2 or above	
LDL or Non-HDL (mmol/l)	No current recommendation Result used with other risk factors to assess CVD 10-year risk score (see below)	
Triglycerides (mmol/l)	🟩 Less than 1.7 🟨 Less than 2.3	
Total cholesterol/HDL ratio	🟩 Less than 4.0	
Kidney Function: ACR (mg/mmol) eGFR (ml/min)	🟩 Men-less than 2.5 & Women-less than 3.5 🟩 60 or more 🟨 30 to 59 🟥 Less than 30	
Inflammation: CRP (mg/l)	🟩 Less than 5.0	
Liver function: GGT (iu/l)	🟩 Men: 11 - 50 🟩 Women: 7 - 32	
CVD 10-year risk score assessment QRISK2 (%)	🟩 Less than 10 🟨 Between 10 - 20 🟥 More than 20	

Traffic 🟩 National target for good health
Light 🟨 Do I need to take action to improve my health?
Coding 🟥 What could I do to improve my health?